THE FIELD GUIDE TO
F*CKING

THE FIELD GUIDE TO
F*CKING

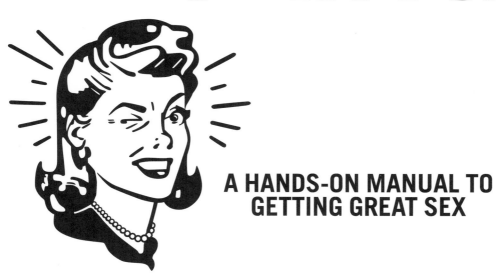

A HANDS-ON MANUAL TO GETTING GREAT SEX

EMILY DUBBERLEY

Author of The Going Down Guide

First published in the USA in 2012 by
Quiver, a member of
Quayside Publishing Group
100 Cummings Center
Suite 406-L
Beverly, MA 01915-6101
www.quiverbooks.com

16 15 14 13 12   1 2 3 4 5

ISBN: 978-1-59233-509-1

Digital edition published in 2012
eISBN: 978-1-61058-398-5

Library of Congress Cataloging-in-Publication Data available

Cover design by Paul Burgess
Illustrations by Robert Brandt

Printed and bound in Singapore

FOR JULIA ARMSTRONG, WHOSE
WISDOM, COMPASSION, AND STRENGTH
HAVE BEEN EDUCATIONAL AND
INSPIRATIONAL.

THANK YOU.

CONTENTS

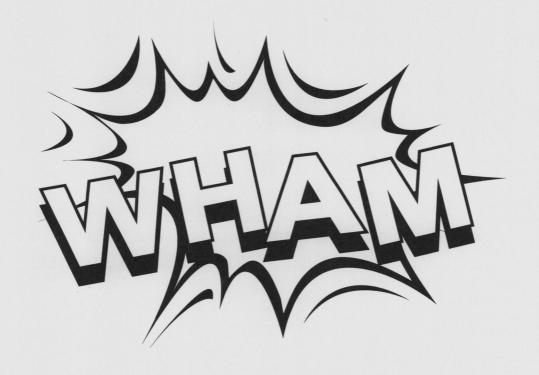

Introduction:

Understanding the Complexities of Coitus

The act of copulation has long attracted keen scholars eager to understand its secrets. Psychologists, neurologists, and doctors have all sought to explain the complex *Homo sapiens* mating ritual. It is also an area of research that attracts millions of lay scholars, with many selflessly conducting exhaustive field studies to hone their own comprehension of the topic.

This text draws on both academic and anecdotal studies to examine every aspect of male-female coitus, presenting a detailed guide to this most valued—and feared—part of human behavior.

When searching for a mate, humans engage in numerous behaviors rarely seen elsewhere in the animal kingdom: using sexual signifiers as base as pointing the fingers toward the genital region or as sophisticated as linguistic trickery to lure a mate; using clothing to indicate sexual preferences (see the eminent report *Short Skirts and Low-Cut Tops*

as a Predictor of Mating Success); and, of course, engaging in the bizarre practices known as oral and manual coitus.

Brave researchers have nobly given their bodies and minds to science in a selfless quest to help the amateur scientist enjoy a more thorough understanding of copulatory habits. However, reading about the act alone is not enough to understand its complexity. Eager scholars should be willing to enter the field themselves, carrying out vigorous and exhaustive studies in order to truly come to grips with the subject.

Gaining research subjects can be an issue for the neophyte student. However, initial research can be conducted on a solo basis, allowing scholars to gain a basic understanding of the area from which to develop their skills. Please ensure that you wash your hands before proceeding to chapter 1.

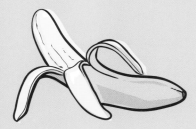

Chapter 1:

Approaching the Field

SURPRISES IN BASIC ANATOMY

The novice scholar is all too often prone to rush into advanced fieldwork without covering those all-important first bases. Before it is possible to master the complexities of the most intimate interpersonal interaction known to man, students first need to get to know an individual who will give 100 percent accurate feedback.

Finding a suitably honest study partner requires a more developed skill set than the average beginner will be able to muster. However, self-study has long been a part of the scientific tradition, and it allows research to commence without any requirement for complex background work.

Ensuring laboratory conditions are hygienic is essential. Use alcohol wipes or soap and water to clean the hands, making sure that all soap is thoroughly removed before exploration commences.

SOLO EXPLORATION: A HANDS-ON APPROACH

Although keen students may have practiced amateur exploration of the genital region, the objective of this investigation is not climax, but rather comprehension. Understanding the way in which one's own genitalia is structured, and the anomalies that may be found in each individual, opens the scholar's mind to differences with potential research partners.

Although physical sensation may serve as a distraction to the undisciplined scholar, students who are keen to graduate with the very highest honors should ensure that they pay equal attention to the visual aspect of exploration. This is innately easier for male students, but female scholars can easily complete the assignment with the addition of a hand mirror. Shaving the pubis prior to exploration may also assist in categorizing the genitals, allowing an unfettered view of the area.

Should any arousal occur during the exploratory process, simply remove your hands until the danger of climax has passed. Alternatively, you may use the masturbatory process as a method of gaining extra credit by observing the effects of arousal, plateau, and climax upon the genital region.

Should you choose this option, pay particular attention to any genital sensitivity once climax has been reached, as an awareness of one's own sensitivities at every stage of coitus will prove useful when proceeding to research with a study partner.

Contraindications

The sexual scholar is often stigmatized. As such, it is essential to conduct these experiments in private. Do not inform your next of kin. Ensure that the laboratory is sealed to prevent any interruptions. Should the experiment carry danger of extreme vocal response, with no soundproofed study area available, consider investing in a gag or biting a pillow.

ESTABLISHING PHYSICAL CONSTRUCTION OF THE GENITAL REGION: THE FEMALE SEX ORGANS

GENERAL ANATOMY

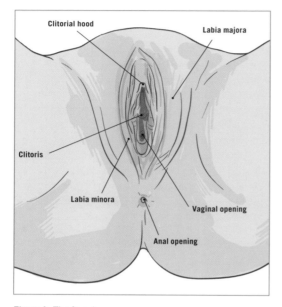

Figure 1: The female sex organs

MONS. This fatty area of tissue above the clitoris offers the willing student an excellent starting position when initiating manual congress. By stimulating the mons with a cupped hand, the clitoral hood retracts, giving easy access to the most densely nerve-packed area of the female genitalia.

CLITORAL HOOD. The clitoral hood, the female equivalent to the foreskin, protects the delicate clitoris from the worst excesses of manhandling. It generally retracts as a woman becomes more aroused. Do not assume direct stimulation of the clitoral tip is always welcome. Test the area gently before proceeding further.

An understanding of the role of the clitoral hood in sexual congress may help a scholar receive the ultimate accolade of multiple orgasms. However, this is a significant challenge that researchers should not embark upon without a comprehensive initial study of the area, because of the myriad variations in clitoral response. Some students may find direct stimulation of the clitoris creates a painful rather than pleasurable response from the recipient.

CLITORIS. Although the clitoris has been the topic of much debate (see *Negative Attitudes Toward Asking for Directions: Male Clitoral Issues Explained*), it is an area worthy of extensive study. Situated above the vagina and labia minora, it responds to stimulation by swelling. Studies have found that each clitoris differs in its response to stimulation (see *Two Hundred Women and Every One Different: Why Men Are Screwed*). Some respond to firm pressure. Others are best approached with a light touch. Vibration can be anathema or the ideal. More research into this area is required.

VAGINA. Although the vagina tends to attract the most interest from the male student, it is often ignored by the female student in favor of the clitoris and secondary erogenous zones. The vagina is less sensitive than the clitoris, meaning penetration alone is unlikely to lead to female climax. However, by understanding this area thoroughly, the female student can increase her climactic chances.

STUDIES HAVE FOUND THAT EACH CLITORIS DIFFERS IN ITS RESPONSE TO STIMULATION (SEE *TWO HUNDRED WOMEN AND EVERY ONE DIFFERENT: WHY MEN ARE SCREWED*).

Tightness of the vagina varies from woman to woman. In addition, some women have smoother vaginas than others, possibly as a result of muscle tone. All vaginas are elastic and expand during arousal. However, different women respond differently to the feeling of being stretched. Some enjoy it, while others find it extremely uncomfortable. This is a key area to focus on during self-stimulation, as it will aid in the process of finding an ideal genital match.

Also, it is worth exploring the absence or presence of a G-spot (see G-Spot), as understanding this elusive area can often open the door to vaginal penetration–induced climax. In addition, it also gives key indicators as to the perfect penis for personal enjoyment.

Note for the male scholar: Regardless of the lack of nerve endings, the psychological sense of well-being that many female scholars get from vaginal penetration by a partner should not be overlooked. However, it is best not to bring this up should a female partner complain about any lack of satisfaction during coitus.

CERVIX. The cervix is located at the back of the vagina and feels round when touched with a finger. Approach the cervix gently because some women find cervical stimulation painful; others find it adds an exciting edge to coitus. Should manual dexterity be limited, students may find it easier to stimulate the cervix, for research purposes, using a vibrator. The resourceful student can gain extra credit by opting for a vibrator with a curved tip because this can also be used to locate the G-spot.

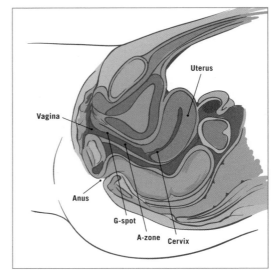

Figure 2: Internal female anatomy: identifying the hidden intricacies of the female genital region

Note for the male scholar: As a women becomes more aroused, her cervix tilts back to ease penetration. However, deep penetration will still stimulate the cervix. This should not automatically be perceived as positive (see *Harder, Faster, Deeper, Ouch!—A Qualitative Analysis of Maximum Penetration*).

G-SPOT. Rumors of the G-spot's extinct status are rife. However, many female lay scholars claim to have a thorough understanding of this unusual anatomical anomaly. Found between one-third and two-thirds the way up the vagina, on the front wall, toward the stomach rather than the anus, the G-spot is most easily stimulated with a curved sexual stimulation device or crooked finger beckoning upward. New research suggests that the G-spot is linked to female ejaculation. The researchers were required to wear raincoats.

NEW RESEARCH SUGGESTS THAT THE G-SPOT IS LINKED TO FEMALE EJACULATION. THE RESEARCHERS WERE REQUIRED TO WEAR RAINCOATS.

A-ZONE. Created on a day when women's magazines were running out of topics to write about, the A-zone is found on the back wall of the vagina, a bit higher than where the G-spot is on the front wall. Correctly stimulated, it will cause strong vaginal contractions.

Note for the male scholar: Incorrect stimulation of the A-zone can lead to a slap.

VARIATIONS IN FEMALE GENITAL STRUCTURE

Whereas the discussed criteria can be applied to female genitalia in general, a high degree of variation exists between individual genitals. They can differ not only in appearance, but also in sensitivity, size of constituent parts, and of course, levels of hygiene and grooming. All these factors can influence the way the genitals should be approached.

Later assignments will cover specific sexual techniques to suit the genitalia with which students are confronted. However, it is also worth categorizing one's own genitalia to assist with identifying the ideal genital match. Ideal genital pairings should take into account all of the following factors, but they are merely a guide from which you can make your own ideal genital match assessment based on the exact criteria of your own genitals.

Size and Shape of the Clitoris

The clitoris varies massively in size, from a barely visible dot to a miniature penis. In July 1992, *The Journal of Obstetrics and Gynaecology* published a study based on the examination of two hundred women. It found:

- The average crosswise width of the clitoral glans was 3.4 mm (0.13 inch), with a range of 2.4 to 4.4 mm (0.09 to 0.17 inch).
- The average lengthwise width was 5.1 mm (0.20 inch), with a range of 3.7 to 6.5 mm (0.15 to 0.26 inch).
- The average total clitoral length including the glans and body was 16.0 mm (0.63 inch), with a range of 11.7 to 20.3 mm (0.46 to 0.80 inch).
- The clitoral index (CI), which took into account the clitoral glans's lengthwise and crosswise widths, was 18.5 mm^2 (0.03 $inch^2$).

The study found no correlation between weight, height, or use of oral contraceptives and clitoral size. However, women who had given birth had "significantly larger measurements."

To establish the size of your clitoris, use a hand mirror and a piece of dental floss. Stretch the dental floss carefully over the area first widthwise, then lengthwise, being careful not to press the floss down on the sensitive clitoris, and measure the floss each time.

Repeat the study after applying stimulation using manual or battery-assisted pleasuring techniques. The clitoris engorges during arousal, and knowing the level of difference between flaccid and erect states can inform your decision about optimal coital positions.

Next, move on to observation using the hand mirror. The shape of the clitoris varies from woman to woman. Although increased androgen levels in the womb can lead to a more phallic structure, this is perfectly natural. Racial heritage may also play a part in the shape of the genitalia, which can lead to insecurity in non-Caucasian women as most anatomy books (and indeed, adult media) are based on Caucasian ideals.

APPROACHING THE FIELD

A FUNCTIONAL CLITORIS IS THE GATEKEEPER OF ORGASM AND, AS SUCH, IS TO BE APPRECIATED REGARDLESS OF ITS SIZE.

A clitoris that projects more than is traditionally depicted is nothing to be ashamed of and, indeed, lends itself more easily to stimulation during penetrative coitus. While you are making a note of your clitoral size and shape, observe the color of the clitoris both before and after stimulation. It will darken as it becomes aroused because of the rush of blood to the area. This is purely academic but allows the keen student to gain a vivid picture of her sexual anatomy during arousal.

Regardless of the size or shape of the clitoris, pleasure can be gained through correct stimulation (assuming there are no medical disorders, including psychological, to take into consideration).

Although some students may feel insecure as a result of their findings, it is worth bearing in mind that there is no such thing as "normal." A functional clitoris is the gatekeeper of orgasm and, as such, is to be appreciated regardless of its size.

SMALL CLITORIS. Although a small clitoris may be hard to find, this is easily rectified with thorough communication. Masturbating in front of a partner will easily identify the area that he should focus on. In addition, this helps build a bond between partners and can act as precoital stimulation for the male.

Should clitoral stimulation prove difficult through coitus, providing the male with a vibrating cock ring may help increase stimulation. In addition, manual stimulation of your own clitoris during coitus will help increase the chance of satisfaction. Further, mating with a male who has an insensitive penis can prolong the act, which may be beneficial.

A small clitoris may be more easily stimulated with a large penis, because this will stretch the clitoral hood over the clitoris, offering indirect stimulation. However, this choice should be balanced against clitoral sensitivity, because a small but sensitive clitoris may find such stimulation too intense.

Cunnilingus is encouraged, as the tongue is considerably more sensitive than the fingers and, as such, may be able to identify the appropriate area more easily.

Ideal match: large penis, mildly insensitive or insensitive penis

MEDIUM CLITORIS. A medium-size clitoris should be relatively easy to stimulate manually, orally, and during coitus. Optimum positions include missionary, woman on top, and coital alignment technique (also known as CAT). See chapter 5, Coitus Complexitus Improvedicus, for further information.

As with a small clitoris, additional stimulation may be gained by using a vibrating cock ring during coitus. Solo stimulation is also encouraged. Cunnilingus, too, offers many joys.

Ideal match: medium or large penis

LARGE CLITORIS. A woman blessed with a large clitoris is likely to find coitus more pleasurable than her less endowed sisters. A large clitoris can be stimulated in most sexual positions, either through the rubbing of the male's shaft against the clitoris during the missionary position or through manual stimulation from either party during rear-entry sexual intercourse. Cunnilingus can incorporate a greater variety of techniques (see chapter 4, Understanding Oral-Genital Congress), as can manual-genital contact.

In addition, locating the clitoris may be easier for the unsophisticated male, making such females ideal for the neophyte student. However, it is not deemed polite to question a woman about her genital dimensions until you have had at least three dates. Seeking pictorial evidence is also unlikely to garner the desired result. Instead, it is simply a case of being grateful for whatever you're given, a state that many males will already be familiar with.

Ideal match: small or medium penis, sensitive or responsive penis

Sensitivity of the Clitoris

The clitoris contains 8,000 nerve endings; compare this to 4,000 nerve endings in the penis, which are obviously spread over a wider area. As such, women are capable of experiencing more intense sensations than men, assuming the male is capable of locating this nerve-rich area in the first place.

It should be noted that the clitoral area is inclined to be sensitive as a result of this nerve density, so the approach should be tailored accordingly. Indeed, biology may well preclude hard, fast stimulation, as desired by the majority of males, and call for gentler treatment. Any male who is sexually sophisticated enough to acknowledge males and females require a different approach is liable to score highly. However, levels of clitoral sensitivity do vary among women.

To test your sensitivity, start by stroking the clitoris with a lubricated finger, through the clitoral hood. If this causes no discomfort, retract the clitoral hood gently by pressing the heel of the hand into the pubic mound. Now touch the tip of the clitoris directly. Stop if it is remotely painful.

To further explore levels of sensitivity, use a bullet vibrator with multiple speed settings. Start with the mildest setting and repeat this experiment. Repeat as you cycle through the settings, stopping when direct stimulation becomes uncomfortable.

An extremely sensitive clitoris will find all but manual touch through the clitoral hood uncomfortable. A sensitive clitoris will generally be able to cope with mild vibrator settings applied through the clitoral hood. A responsive clitoris will respond eagerly to mid-level stimulation, while a mildly insensitive clitoris may require higher vibrator settings. An extremely insensitive clitoris may require the highest vibrator settings or retraction of the clitoral hood.

Again, none of these categorizations are right or wrong, desirable or undesirable. However, by understanding your level of clitoral sensitivity, you can tailor sexual activities to achieve the most pleasurable results.

EXTREMELY SENSITIVE CLITORIS. An extremely sensitive clitoris can limit sexual activity. However, with appropriate treatment, it is still entirely possible to have enjoyable sexual interactions. Manual sex should not be attempted without lubricant. In addition, it is recommended that you place your hand either underneath or on top of your partner's as he stimulates you so you can control the amount of pressure that is used.

Cunnilingus should only be attempted if the male is extremely clean-shaven and should focus more on lapping than suction (see chapter 4, Understanding Oral-Genital Congress, for further information).

Coitus should ideally avoid clitoral contact. Therefore, rear-entry positions are likely to be the most effective.

Ideal Match: small penis, sensitive penis

SENSITIVE CLITORIS. A sensitive clitoris may encounter issues similar to an extremely sensitive clitoris. However, coitus may be possible in a greater variety of positions. Woman on top is ideal, as it allows the female to control the level of clitoral stimulation by angling her body appropriately. Manual contact should only be attempted with lubricant, and again, a level of guidance is recommended. Cunnilingus should be extremely gentle and suction should be avoided.

Ideal match: small penis, sensitive penis

RESPONSIVE CLITORIS. A responsive clitoris can be stimulated in multiple coital positions. In addition, most cunnilingus and manual stimulation techniques can be used.

Ideal match: responsive penis

MILDLY INSENSITIVE CLITORIS. A mildly insensitive clitoris may require the addition of a vibrating cock ring or manually controlled bullet vibrator to ensure coitus results in climax. Similarly, toys should be incorporated into manual and oral-genital congress. Additional stimulation may be required in the form of talking dirty or watching an adult film. Furthermore, women (and some men) often respond to reading erotic literature or hearing it read out loud by a partner. Note that these activities should not be saved purely for females with a mildly insensitive clitoris but are more likely to be required in this case.

Ideal match: large penis, mildly insensitive or extremely insensitive penis

EXTREMELY INSENSITIVE CLITORIS. As with a mildly insensitive clitoris, the extremely insensitive clitoris may require additional mental stimulation in order to rouse it. CAT with the male wearing a vibrating cock ring offers the optimum level of clitoral stimulation during coitus (see chapter 5, Coitus Complexitus Improvedicus). Oral and manual techniques should involve toys in addition to the hands or tongue.

Ideal match: large penis, mildly insensitive or extremely insensitive penis

Symmetry and the Genitals

Although symmetrical genitalia are often presented as the ideal, in reality, almost every part of the body is nonsymmetrical: One foot is often larger than the other; one breast is generally larger than the other; and many people have more developed muscles on either their left or their right side. Therefore, applying such criteria to the genitalia is not worthy of consideration. It is mentioned purely to dispel the myth of "perfect" genitals.

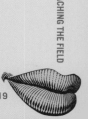

Size and Shape of Labia

As with the clitoris, the labia can vary in size and shape. Although adult films frequently depict small and neat heart-shaped inner and outer labia, many women have wrinkled labia with a less symmetrical shape. The labia minora may protrude below the level of the labia majora, which, again, can lead to insecurity in the female species. However, unless there is any medical reason for surgery, this is not something to be concerned about. Indeed, some cultures throughout history have idealized larger labia, leading to practices that aim to stretch the labia more extremely. This is not recommended without medical supervision.

As far back as 1932, American obstetrician Robert Latou Dickinson reported wide variation in labial size. Whereas 87 percent of women had labia that were 2 cm (0.75 inch) in width, he claimed to have examined a woman's labia minora that measured 7.5 cm (3 inches) on each side, 15 cm (6 inches) tip to tip when spread open, and almost 11.5 cm (4.5 inches), or 23 cm (9 inches) tip to tip, in length when placed under moderate tension. He further reported five cases that measured between 5 and 7.5 cm (2 and 3 inches) when spread open.

To measure your labia, use the same floss technique as for clitoral measurement. First measure the outer labia, then the inner labia. Although the labia have less bearing on coitus than the clitoris does, extended labia may be wrapped around the penis prior to intercourse for an exciting variation on standard masturbation, which offers both parties equal sexual pleasure.

In addition to size and level of protuberance, the labia can vary in shape, with some being more curled than others. As the labia fill with blood, these folds stretch out, meaning that this has little bearing on coitus. However, getting to know every area of your genitals allows for thorough comprehension of the subject.

Indeed, all studies into genitalia perfection to date, based on analyzing visual depictions in adult media, have had to be curtailed, as the researchers ran out of tissues. Further field studies in lap-dancing clubs also had to be curtailed because of researcher bias (see *Boobs, Bums, Legs, or Something in Between: An Analysis of Male Sexual Desires*, by Hermitage Shank, MD).

Depth of Vagina

Although little research has been conducted in the area, popular opinion asserts that the vagina is generally 7.5 to 10 cm (3 to 4 inches) deep in a nonaroused state and stretches during arousal to accommodate the penis. However, some women prefer deeper penetration than others, regardless of the level to which the vagina easily stretches (see *How Deep Is Your Love? In Search of the Perfect Pounding: An Ethnographic Approach*, by Jilly Love, MD).

To test your capacity for penetration, start by stimulating yourself to near climax. Then use a phallic vibrator to penetrate yourself to optimum levels. This may take some time, and indeed, gradually increasing the depth of penetration will be more effective than aiming for the cervix at first thrust. Once optimal penetration has been identified, measure the depth to which the vibrator has penetrated. This gives an indication of the ideal length of penis for your vagina, though you should take into account girth and shape as well.

While conducting this test, it is worth checking the cervix's sensitivity to pressure. Gently nudge the vibrator against the cervix, only increasing pressure if it creates a pleasurable sensation. If the cervix is sensitive, this is worth considering when choosing a position for coitus (see chapter 5, Coitus Complexitus Improvedicus).

To establish the desired girth of a partner, either invest in inexpensive toys of different girths or buy an inflatable dildo. This allows you to vary the size during

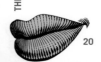

use. Again, once you have identified the optimal size, measure the toy to take a note of your findings. Should the girth be larger than the majority of males, you may wish to consider using toys in addition to a phallus during coitus. This should be introduced on the basis of vibration rather than size to ensure that the male study partner remains motivated.

SHALLOW VAGINA. A woman with a shallow vagina may find coitus uncomfortable in rear-entry positions. Instead, missionary position is recommended, with the legs flat on the bed to minimize the depth of penetration. Woman-on-top positions are also good because they put the woman in control. Manual stimulation should take a second place to oral stimulation, as a woman with a shallow vagina may well be less likely to crave deep penetration as part of the precoital routine.

Ideal match: small penis, mildly sensitive or extremely sensitive penis

MEDIUM VAGINA. This allows for a range of most sexual positions and techniques. However, should penetration become uncomfortable, take steps to minimize discomfort when choosing positions (see Shallow Vagina).

Ideal match: medium penis, responsive penis

DEEP VAGINA. A woman with a deep vagina is liable to enjoy "porn star sex" more than a woman who has less depth. Rear-entry positions offer the greatest potential for maximum penetration. In addition, if the female arches her back, this is likely to increase the intensity. Approaching from the rear with a vibrator or fingers during manual stimulation is also likely to be well received.

Ideal match: large penis, mildly insensitive or extremely insensitive penis

Tightness of the Vagina

The vagina varies in tightness depending on both individual biology and muscular definition. Although a "tight" vagina is held up as the physical ideal, this is a stereotype that doesn't always ring true: a man with a large phallus may find penetration uncomfortable, and a tight vagina may also be difficult to penetrate if the male isn't extremely hard.

Further, the medical condition of vaginismus, which causes the vagina to tighten up to such a level that it is impenetrable, can negate the opportunity for coitus altogether. Should this condition be in evidence, it is essential to seek medical care, which can involve both physical and psychological treatment.

However, medical issues aside, as a general rule, more toned vaginal muscles will allow for greater friction during coitus, which can enhance satisfaction for both parties involved. Good muscular control will also allow the female to flex her muscles during copulation, which can add pleasure to the experience. As such, it is worth including vaginal toning as part of a general exercise routine. This is particularly important if a woman has given birth, as the birthing process can lead to vaginal slackening.

Kegel exercises, named after the doctor who created them, entail flexing and releasing the vaginal muscles. There are numerous pelvic toning devices available to help with this process, some of which are simply weights to be held in the vagina; others work on the basis of resistance, in a similar way to thigh toners but on a considerably smaller scale.

Alternatively, the female scholar may opt to first identify the muscles by inserting a finger into the vagina and flexing her vaginal muscles until they contract around the finger or by sitting on the toilet and attempting to hold back the flow during urination. However, the latter technique should be used purely as a means of identifying which set of muscles to exercise because regular attempts to control the flow of urine in this way may lead to kidney infections.

SOME SCHOLARS MAY BE UNABLE TO FIND THE G-SPOT AT ALL. THIS WILL **NOT** COST YOU ANY CREDITS.

Once the muscles have been identified, the female student should exercise daily, with a minimum of ten contractions. First clench the muscles, and then hold them for a count of ten before slowly letting the muscles relax back to the resting position. Not only will this exercise help increase vaginal tone, it will also boost blood flow to the area, which can have a beneficial effect upon both the quantity and the quality of orgasms. Rapid flexing of the Kegel muscles during coitus can elicit a positive response.

TIGHT VAGINA. Although the tight vagina is often idealized because it offers the greatest level of friction, it may limit congress with a well-endowed male. Lubricant is near essential unless the woman produces large amounts of natural juices. In addition, though it may seem counterintuitive, regular Kegel exercises will help improve muscle tone, making it easier to accept a larger penis. Bearing down with the muscles may ease entry.

Should penetration prove difficult, rear-entry sex positions may ease the way, particularly if the female spreads her legs widely. Woman-on-top positions will also be beneficial, particularly if the tightness is caused partly by nerves, as the woman can control the pace. Extended foreplay sessions should help relax the vagina, making it looser and easier to penetrate.

Ideal match: small penis, mildly sensitive or extremely sensitive penis

MEDIUM VAGINA. A regular vagina will comfortably accept all but the largest penis. Should a small-membered man be unable to provide satisfaction, the vagina can be tightened by the women crossing her legs during doggy-style sex. Alternatively, the legs can be crossed during spooning, or first raised and then crossed to the side of the body during missionary-style sex. Conversely, the vagina can be loosened to accommodate a larger male by stretching the women's legs wide. Most precoital arousal techniques should meet with a positive response.

Ideal match: medium penis, responsive penis

LOOSE VAGINA. Though a loose vagina may not provide enough friction for a male with a small phallus, it can be a blessing in disguise for a well-endowed man, offering ease of penetration. Foreplay techniques may be improved with the addition of vibrators or dildos to provide a "filling" sensation.

Ideal match: large penis, mildly insensitive or extremely insensitive penis

The G-Spot Location, Sensitivity, and Penetration Preferences

The female scholar should attempt to find her G-spot. This may be done manually with a curved finger, but will be considerably easier with a specially designed toy. Start by initiating stimulation, then, once climax is near, insert the G-spot toy slowly and twist it around until you find an area that responds differently than the rest of the vagina. This response may be pleasurable. Alternatively, it may cause the urge to urinate.

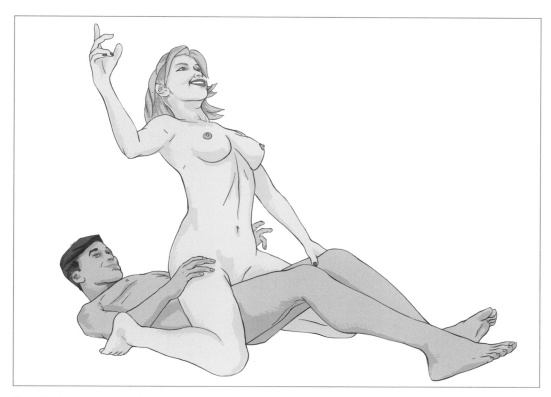

Figure 3: Try stimulating the G-spot through the reverse cowgirl position.

Some scholars may be unable to find the G-spot at all. This will not cost you any credits. Understanding whether you have a G-spot and, if so, how it responds can be a valuable indicator of both ideal sexual positions and manual or oral-genital stimulation techniques.

PLEASURABLE G-SPOT. Should a woman enjoy G-spot stimulation, rear-entry positions are recommended. Similarly, approaching from behind when initiating manual or oral-genital congress should garner a positive response.

To enhance the missionary position, the woman should raise her legs until the penis is angled directly into her G-spot. Reverse cowgirl, in which the female straddles the male while facing his feet, is another surefire way to stimulate the G-spot.

Ideal match: large penis

UNCOMFORTABLE G-SPOT. Should G-spot stimulation prove uncomfortable, rear-entry positions should be avoided in favor of missionary or woman on top. Spooning and flat doggy offer the shallowest penetration of all rear-entry positions, should you wish to experiment with alternative approaches.

Ideal match: small penis

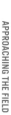

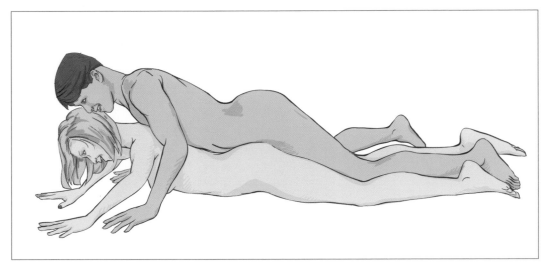

Figure 4: The flat doggy position offers the least depth of penetration for women with an over-sensitive G-spot.

CATEGORIZING THE FEMALE GENITALS

Once all measurements and readings have been taken, create a chart of your unique sexual blueprint. This is for your own study purposes and will not be graded by anyone else, unless you choose to share it for extra communication credits. However, the chart should be used to refer back to congress of any kind, to ensure that optimal precoital arousal techniques are used and the ideal position for coitus is chosen (subject to compatibility with your research partner's blueprint).

In addition, make a note of all potentially compatible male members to create a blueprint for your ideal genital match. Should different aspects of your genital structure require different types of phallus, either use your common sense to identify your preference or experiment with all variations until the ideal is found.

Should you have a network of females who are also inclined to study The Field Guide to F*cking, you may find it useful to compare charts. This will help you gain a more in-depth understanding of the differences in sexual formation and can also prove a useful bonding exercise among female friends. However, do not progress to physical comparisons unless you have an extreme affinity with your fellow researcher or mutual bicurious tendencies.

ESTABLISHING PHYSICAL CONSTRUCTION OF THE GENITAL REGION: THE MALE SEX ORGANS

GENERAL ANATOMY

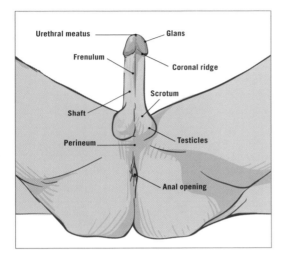

Figure 5: The male sex organs

GLANS. Also known as the head, the glans is one of the most sensitive parts of the penis. As such, initial exploration of the area should be tentative to avoid accidental ejaculation. Note the way in which the glans swells and darkens in color during stimulation. Consider the relative difference between the circumference of the glans and the shaft, as this can have a significant effect on preferential positions for coitus.

URETHRAL MEATUS. The man's ejaculate shoots through the urethral meatus. Many renegade male students have experimented with penetration of the urethral meatus using flowers, chopsticks, or in extreme cases, another penis. This is not recommended and can be extremely dangerous.

Note for female scholars: Sadly, the urethral meatus lacks any stop function. As such, many a neophyte female student has suffered from unfortunate consequences in believing a man who promises not to ejaculate in her oral cavity. Sticking the tongue down the meatus will not halt the flow.

FORESKIN. The foreskin offers a protective coat for the glans. Said coat is removed from many men at an early age, thus exposing the glans and removing the penis's ability to self-lubricate (see *Lubricant Sales in the Cut and Uncut Man*). Circumcision may also decrease sensitivity. Experimenting with different lubricants, including stimulating and warming ones, may help enhance sensation. Although different women have different preferences, undergoing foreskin removal at the behest of a woman should be taken no more seriously than a request to have a leg amputated.

CORONAL RIDGE. This is the ridge around the bottom of the glans. Many have tried to understand its purpose (see *Inhibiting Manual Slippage During Male Masturbation: A Physiological Study*). What is known is that the corona responds particularly positively to stimulation. Avoiding direct stimulation of this area may help slow climax.

FRENULUM. Central in the coronal ridge is the frenulum, a string of membrane that attaches the glans to the shaft. This is also a key area of sensitivity for many men and, as such, should be explored to better understand the stimulatory options available.

SHAFT. Forming the bulk of the penis, the shaft swells during arousal. It has been posited that the shaft evolved to help ensure that the male ego remain controlled by creating numerous insecurities about its requisite dimensions. The thicker member is often vaunted but only if teamed with length. Curvature may also lead to paranoia. However, assuming medical issues are ruled out, the confident student in possession of a curved shaft can use this to enhance coitus, particularly with regard to G-spot stimulation.

VARIATIONS IN MALE GENITAL STRUCTURE

Size of the Penis

According to a 2003 study of 5,000 men (source: www.the-penis.com), the average erect penis is 15 cm (5.9 inches) long and 12.7 cm (5 inches) in girth. However, modern adult films tend to focus on genitalia of unusually large size. This can cause many male students to feel lacking.

Although the average penis in a pornographic feature is generally a minimum of 20.3 cm (8 inches), this does not necessarily enhance sex or provide a female ideal. Indeed, it is worth considering that the majority of viewers of adult films are male and, as such, depictions therein are more likely to cater to a masculine than a feminine ideal. A small penis is still perfectly capable of providing a woman with erotic satisfaction, as the majority of nerves in the vagina are within the first 7.5 to 10 cm (3 to 4 inches) of the vaginal canal.

Conversely, if a male feels blessed to have a member of extreme size, this does not mean that he should ignore chapters on manual and oral-genital congress and move immediately to coitus. Indeed, this common mistake has led many well-endowed men to fail in their endeavors to make a partner reach climax.

SMALL PENIS. Although a small penis may lead to male insecurity, it can be optimal for coitus with a woman who has a shallow or tight vagina. In addition, many sex acts are considerably easier with a small phallus: notably, deep throat and anal coitus.

Although a small penis is less than ideal for G-spot stimulation, this can be rectified by choosing rear-entry sex positions (see chapter 5, Coitus Complexitus Improvedicus). Should a man with a small phallus couple with a woman who has a preference for deep penetration, there is no reason that toys cannot be used in addition to coitus. Further, using a cock ring will help the penis achieve maximum hardness, and opting for a vibrating version will generally help speed the female's climax, too.

Anecdotal evidence suggests that women are less concerned about size than men may suspect, as long as manual and oral-genital skills are suitably honed.

Ideal match: shallow vagina, tight vagina, sensitive or extremely sensitive clitoris

MEDIUM PENIS. A medium penis can still lead to feelings of inadequacy in a male, due to the common depictions of male members in adult films. However, as with a small penis, a medium-size penis is generally preferable to a large one for both oral and anal coitus.

Shaving the pubic region will make a phallus appear larger. However, appearance is less important than performance. Should deeper penetration be desired, opting for rear-entry positions will help. Changing the angle of entry by urging a female partner to lift her hips or place her ankles around the male's neck will also increase the depth of penetration.

Ideal match: medium vagina, responsive clitoris

Measuring Criteria for Optimal Genital Sizing

It is anecdotally understood that many male lay scholars have engaged in measuring the penis for recreational entertainment. However, this is commonly undertaken without utilizing the scientific method and can lead to gross distortions in data.

To correctly measure the penis, measurements should be taken from the base of the penis to the tip of the glans. This requires measuring along the upper rather than the lower side of the penis.

Males opting to measure the underside of the penis often start at the anus to enhance their statistics. However, this is false accounting that is sure to be judged harshly should such measurements be made public. Once the phallus is utilized for sexual activity, the genuine size will become all too easily apparent.

To correctly measure the girth of the penis, simply take a piece of string and place it around the center of the shaft, cutting it to size, then measure the piece of string. The particularly rigorous student can also measure around the underside of the glans and the base of the shaft, and then average the results. However, using the first method should give a reasonable approximation of the general circumference.

Measuring the penis in both flaccid and erect states will help ensure that the male student has optimal data with which to find a perfect genital match.

Note: The size of a flaccid penis bears little relation to the size of the same member once erect, and men who appear to have radically different penile dimensions when flaccid may well have identically sized members once erect. This phenomena is colloquially referred to as being either a "shower" or a "grower."

LARGE PENIS. Although a man with a large member may feel blessed, do remember that a partner will need to be more lubricated to receive such a phallus. As such, it is essential to spend at least twenty minutes on foreplay to ensure that the cervix tilts back, easing penetration. Additional lubricant may also be required to ensure that entry is not uncomfortable.

A large phallus is generally more effective for G-spot stimulation. However, rear-entry positions may be painful for some women, and rigorous sexual activity may lead to cervical or vaginal bruising. If a female study partner is nervous about the dimensions of the phallus, woman-on-top positions may provide the optimal solution.

Should deep throat be a preference, it is worth finding a partner with a well-trained gag reflex. Under no circumstance should the well-endowed man place his hand on a lover's head during oral sex unless he has been expressly asked to do so.

Ideal match: deep vagina, loose vagina, insensitive or extremely insensitive clitoris

Sensitivity of the Penis

As with female anatomy, male genitalia can vary greatly in terms of sensitivity. While men tend to prefer more rigorous and rapid stimulation of the genital region than women, this can be painful if a male has a particularly sensitive member.

To test sensitivity, masturbate the penis to erection. Now see how long it takes to ejaculate from this point. If climax can be attained within one minute or stimulation is painful, you have an extremely sensitive penis. If climax takes two minutes, your penis is sensitive. If it is relatively easy to last five minutes, you have a responsive penis. If it takes eight minutes, you have a mildly insensitive penis. If it takes ten minutes or longer, you have an extremely insensitive penis.

Also consider the amount of time it takes you to reach climax during coitus. Research shows the average male lasts around seven minutes from penetration to climax. A figure that's significantly higher or lower than this will give a clear indication as to the sensitivity of your penis.

As with the clitoris, the sensitivity of the penis can vary over time, and a responsive phallus may become extremely sensitive after an extended sex session. A saltwater bath will speed healing time in cases of extreme chafing.

EXTREMELY SENSITIVE PENIS. If a male has an extremely sensitive penis, it may lead to premature ejaculation. However, this can be easily rectified with the use of thick or "delay" prophylactics. The latter contain anaesthetizing gel that should be washed off after use, should oral coitus be desired, as otherwise it may numb the tongue of a lover and tastes unpleasant.

To further assist with prolonging coitus to ensure mutual satisfaction, foreplay should be kept to a minimum for the male but maximized for the female prior to penetration. Should the penis be so sensitive as to be limited to one ejaculation per session, it is worth ensuring that the female partner is fully satisfied prior to commencing coitus.

Further, fellatio may be limited unless the female partner is willing to receive her sexual satisfaction using alternative methods to coitus.

Ideal match: loose vagina, sensitive or extremely sensitive clitoris

SENSITIVE PENIS. As with the extremely sensitive penis, a male with a sensitive penis may be more likely to ejaculate quickly. Using thick condoms may help, but if this reduces sensation to excessive levels, it may be easier to opt for frequent changes of sexual position and technique as a way of prolonging coitus.

One advantage of a sensitive penis is that the speedy ejaculation that may work to a man's detriment during coitus can be seen as a positive advantage during oral or anal coitus.

Ideal match: loose vagina, sensitive or extremely sensitive clitoris

RESPONSIVE PENIS. A responsive penis will generally last for as long as a partner requires (within reason) without premature ejaculation. It also allows for greater scope in terms of stimulation, as there are few standard activities that are ruled out.

Ideal match: medium vagina, responsive clitoris

MILDLY INSENSITIVE PENIS. A mildly insensitive penis may require more oral or manual stimulation prior to coitus to ensure a suitable level of arousal for ejaculation during the act of coitus. Using the hands in addition to the mouth during oral congress will help speed arousal. Lubricant may be required to avoid chafing during extended periods of stimulation or coitus.

Ideal match: tight vagina, insensitive or extremely insensitive clitoris

EXTREMELY INSENSITIVE PENIS. Males in possession of an extremely insensitive penis may require visual stimulation in addition to manual, oral, or coital stimulation in order to climax. Adult films or an erotic striptease may both prove useful. Stimulating additional areas such as the testicles or prostate gland may also be considered, depending on preference.

As with the mildly insensitive phallus, using lubricant is recommended for extended periods of sexual pleasuring. Warming and cooling lubricants can add an extra frisson to sexual activity, and a vibrating cock ring may also help increase stimulation.

Ideal match: tight vagina, insensitive or extremely insensitive clitoris

Presence or Absence of Foreskin

Circumcision is primarily influenced by culture. Fewer than 20 percent of European males are circumcised, compared to 75 percent of American men. While some claim there are hygiene benefits, there is also clear evidence linking circumcision to psychological and physical trauma. As such, it should only be considered in cases of medical need. Regardless of the ethics of circumcision, it is worth noting that the circumcised and uncircumcised phallus should be handled in different ways.

CIRCUMCISED PENIS. In the circumcised male, chafing may occur after extended periods of manual or coital stimulation. This is because a circumcised penis is liable to self-lubricate to a lesser degree than an uncircumcised phallus. As such, it is essential to have lubricant on hand to ensure that manual

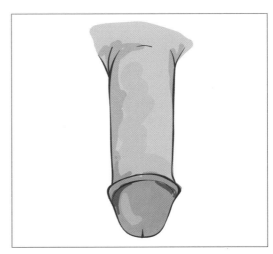

Figure 6: Lubricant is recommended when dealing with a circumcised penis.

stimulation is comfortable, or use saliva as an alternative if the situation is unplanned and there is no lubricant available. Coitus may become more comfortable if a drop of lubricant is put inside the tip of the condom. With unprotected sex, it is worth spending more time stimulating the woman prior to penetration because she will require more of her own lubrication to counterbalance the male's lack of lubrication. Some men find that circumcision leads to insensitivity, particularly around the site of the scar. If so, see the earlier section on dealing with an insensitive penis.

Ideal match: loose vagina if area is sensitive, tight vagina if area is insensitive, insensitive or extremely insensitive clitoris if prolonged intercourse is required for climax

UNCIRCUMCISED PENIS. The uncircumcised penis may be considered unhygienic by some. However, this is a fallacy, as long as the male ensures that he washes underneath the foreskin when attending to his ablutions. The foreskin can be used during both manual and oral pleasuring to enhance the experience. Simply moving the foreskin back and forth over the glans can cause considerable pleasure in a responsive penis, and slipping a tongue underneath the foreskin during oral coitus may also receive a warm reception.

However, if a foreskin is even remotely loose, it is worth removing any rings prior to commencing manual stimulation, to avoid any risk of tearing. Further, should a woman have braces, it may be worth avoiding penetrative oral coitus until they have been removed, instead focusing on licking the area and using manual stimulation methods.

Ideal match: tight vagina, insensitive or extremely insensitive clitoris

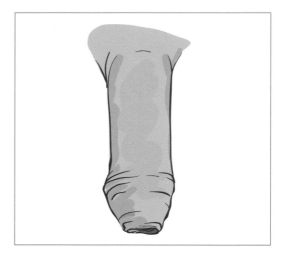

Figure 7: Oral coitus on an uncircumcised penis should be avoided or executed with extreme care if a woman has braces.

Sensitivity of the Testicles

As with the various parts of the penis, the testicles can vary in sensitivity from male to male. Some men enjoy the sensation of tugging, licking, and even gentle nibbling. Others find any stimulation at all to be uncomfortable. A male is likely to have an extremely educated opinion as to his level of testicular sensitivity without any testing required. The female student should note that it is particularly important to request permission before venturing into manual or oral stimulation of this region.

SENSITIVE TESTICLES. All stimulation of sensitive testicles is best avoided. Should a male partner express a willingness to explore, with reservations about his level of sensitivity, use only tongue and focus on licking rather than suction. Trailing the hair over the testicles may also be a treat for a man who is sensitive in this area.

Genitals and Taste/Aroma

In addition to variations in appearance and sensitivity, there can be differences in the way the sexual juices taste. Both genders are affected by diet and lifestyle factors, and generally speaking, the healthier a person is, the more pleasant his or her genitals will taste.

Foods that may negatively affect the taste of sexual juices include asparagus, chili, curry, and fatty foods in general. Recreational use of alcohol and nicotine may add bitterness to the taste. Dehydration can also lead to stronger tasting sexual excretions.

Anecdotal evidence suggests that semen may taste more bitter if a man has not ejaculated for an extended period of time. As such, masturbating before a date in which oral sex is hoped for is polite.

Female sexual juices will vary in taste depending on which stage of the menstrual cycle a woman is in. As menstruation approaches, the juices may taste more metallic because of increased levels of iron in vaginal excretions, and after menstruation, this taste may have an additional "meaty" flavor because of lingering blood. However, assuming that there is no risk of sexually transmitted infections—transmission of which can be exacerbated through exposure to menstrual blood—there is no reason to avoid the area other than preferences of palate.

Male sexual juices are commonly referred to as being bitter or salty. Female sexual juices are commonly referred to as being sweet or sour. The best way to establish how your sexual juices taste is to sample them. That way, you can establish whether a partner is correct should any issues relating to sexual flavor be raised.

Although sexual juices can be masked with the use of flavored lubricants, this hides one of the body's most basic communication methods. Humans are biologically primed to respond to the smell of one another's genitals, in a way that the smell of strawberries or a piña colada can never match.

Even without using artificial means, genitals can also vary in the way they smell. However, if the genitals are clean, they shouldn't smell fishy, cheesy, or in any way unpleasant. Although there are numerous intimate douches on the market, these should be avoided because the vagina self-regulates and using soaps in the genital region can lead to an imbalance in the body's natural pH levels, which, conversely, can lead to noxious odors. Excessive washing of the region can also lead to unpleasant-smelling genitals.

Should a partner's genitals not meet your olfactory satisfaction, this could be an indication of mismatched pheromones and, as such, be considered your body's way of issuing a warning that there may be a biological incompatibility. Although relationships can work between couples who don't appreciate each other's unique taste and smell, these senses are so important to sex that such a union should only be considered in extreme cases.

HUMANS ARE BIOLOGICALLY PRIMED TO RESPOND TO THE SMELL OF ONE ANOTHER'S GENITALS, IN A WAY THAT THE SMELL OF STRAWBERRIES OR A PIÑA COLADA CAN NEVER MATCH.

RESPONSIVE TESTICLES. Responsive testicles can be cupped, licked, and gently sucked. However, they should still be handled with care, as this is a highly sensitive part of the body that bruises easily. Stroking the area may be well received, particularly if the hand then runs down to caress the perineum.

Teabagging, in which the male straddles the female's face and lowers his testicles into her mouth, is a commonly enjoyed method of ball play. It also puts the man in control, allowing him to set the pace, which is ideal if you are new to exploring this region.

INSENSITIVE TESTICLES. Although insensitive testicles can take more handling without discomfort, they should still be treated with respect. Sucking one or both testicles into the mouth may be pleasurable, as may cupping and lightly tugging the testicles during manual stimulation or coitus. Never squeeze the testicles hard, no matter how insensitive they may seem, as this can lead to significant medical issues.

Shape of the Penis

Although one might assume that every phallus is the same, in reality, the shape can vary significantly. The shaft can be highly veined or smooth, while the glans can be of the same circumference as the shaft, taper to a near point, or be significantly larger than the shaft, resulting in a "mushroom head."

A woman with a small vagina may find a tapered penis easier to accept, while a woman with a pleasurably sensitive G-spot may find great satisfaction through skillful use of a mushroom-headed phallus.

Many men also show a curvature of the penis. Should the penis curve only during arousal, it is worth visiting a physician to rule out Peyronie's disease, a disorder in which internal scar tissue causes the penis to bend, particularly if this makes intercourse uncomfortable. However, a mild curvature that doesn't cause any discomfort to either party is nothing to worry about, and may even assist with G-spot stimulation in a genitally compatible female.

Symmetry and the Male Genitalia

Male genitalia are no more symmetrical than that of the female. It is common for one testicle to hang lower than the other, which some claim is designed to make sitting while wearing clothes more comfortable for the male, as the testicles sit on top of each other rather than next to each other.

Similarly, the penis may curve to the left or the right (see Shape of the Penis). As with females, genital symmetry is not something to be concerned about and this section is here simply to shatter any illusions as to its importance.

PHYSICAL ANOMALIES ENCOUNTERED IN THE FIELD

Unlike genetically endowed genital structures, there are optional modifications that may be made to the genitalia. The most common of these is pubic hair styling. However, there are also more niche anomalies, such as jeweled temporary decorations (a technique known as vajazzling and p-jazzling, depending on the gender of the wearer) and genital piercings.

STYLE OF PUBIC HAIR

Generally, women are more likely to amend their natural pubic hair shape because of the dual pressures of women's magazines and depictions of females in adult media. Over the past decade, being hirsute has become ever more frowned upon, and many women feel the pressure to undergo painful waxing to ensure that they are smooth. Further, some women use the stigma attached to pubic hair as a method of self-control, leaving their bodies au naturel on nights when they don't wish to entertain sexual congress.

Regardless of the politics, pubic hair styles can have an impact on sex. However, female students should note that males can be attracted to myriad types of pubic hair and, as such, should style their pubic hair according to their own preference rather than any societal pressures.

FULLY SHAVEN. A fully shaven pubic area allows for easy oral sex without any risk of pubic hairs causing a choking hazard. However, depending on the method of defoliation used, it can also lead to itchy grow-back, ingrown hairs, and heightened sensitivity. The latter can have positive or negative results, either enhancing sex by increasing stimulation or limiting sex because of uncomfortable sensations. If a woman has an extremely sensitive or sensitive clitoris, pubic shaving is not advised.

Some people find the sensation of sliding smooth skin against smooth skin to be pleasurable. However, this requires both genders to fully remove the pubic hair and maintain it regularly, as stubble on the chin can cause particular irritation when rubbing against a shaved mons veneris.

One advantage of removing the pubic hair entirely is that it encourages the utmost exploration, drawing attention to the oft-ignored pubic mound. Using a lubricated hand to massage the entire area shows an appreciation of your partner's grooming habits. Oral exploration is also likely to be well received.

SHAPED. Shaped pubic hair has grown in popularity over the past decade and was popularized (to an extent) when it was featured in the seminal television show *Sex and the City*. The style of shaping chosen can tell you a lot about a potential mate. A heart shape suggests a romantic, for example, and a lightning bolt indicates someone who likes to be perceived as "hot stuff." A woman who goes to the effort of shaping and then dying her pubic hair is clearly someone who doesn't mind setting aside time for all things sexual.

As with fully shaved pubic hair, shaped pubic hair carries a risk of irritation, which may lead to heightened sensitivity. However, by choosing an appropriate pattern, it is possible to minimize chafing. The majority of patterns allow almost as easy access to the entire genital region as shaving in full does. In addition, shaping the pubic hair can add a note of frivolity to proceedings, and can be a sensual way to celebrate Valentine's Day or an anniversary.

TRIMMED. Many women opt for simply trimming the pubic hair into a neat triangle, and possibly removing the hairs on the labia. This has the advantage of allowing easy access to the genital region for oral-genital coitus without the same degree of maintenance required as full pubic shaving. As such, this is a recommended pubic hairstyle for women in long-term relationships, being both practical and tidy.

NATURAL. In allowing the pubic hair to roam free, a woman demonstrates that society's view is of little importance to her. This can suggest that she is more likely to be sexually liberated and willing to explore a diverse range of bedroom habits. However, it may also indicate lack of attention to grooming or present practical issues, particularly related to the act of cunnilingus. Parting the hair manually will make access to the genital region easier.

It is also worth running your fingers through the pubic hair prior to commencing oral activities to help remove any loose hairs and minimize choking hazards. Brushing the pubic hair after bathing is also recommended.

VAJAZZLING AND P-JAZZLING. Decorating the mons with jewels is a relatively recent trend that has been popularized by WAGS (wives and girlfriends of sports stars) and their ilk. This involves fully defoliating the genital region before applying temporary jewels in a decorative manner. Common patterns include hearts, flowers, and national flags. P-jazzling is the male equivalent, though this is an extremely niche activity.

Should a study partner have jeweled nether regions, it suggests attention to detail and a certain desire to shock. However, care should be taken during oral coitus to ensure that no jewels become loose and cause a choking hazard.

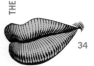

TYPES OF INTIMATE PIERCING AND HOW TO APPROACH THEM

While pubic shaping is relatively common, and vajazzling and p-jazzling are currently fashionable, these are not the only anomalies that may be encountered in the field. Though rare, there are numerous types of intimate piercing that may come as a surprise if one is not suitably briefed.

The lay scholar should be aware that genital piercing is not a recent trend, particularly if he or she wishes to impress an individual who is decorated in such a way. Indeed, texts as ancient as the Kama Sutra have referenced adornments, to the male genitals affixed through a piercing. Further, certain tribes have long used subdermal implants—implants underneath the skin of the penis—to enhance pleasure for female partners.

Although scholars with such an adornments are advised to warn potential mates prior to removing any clothes, there is no reason to feel intimidated.

As a general rule, piercings should be removed prior to using prophylactics to ensure that no accidental tearing of the condom occurs. However, certain piercings, such as subdermal implants, will not cause any damage to the condom and are also thought to enhance sexual pleasure.

Scholars should avoid unprotected sex with a partner who has a fresh piercing, as this can lead to infection and also increases the risk of exposure to sexually transmitted diseases. Once the piercing has healed, unprotected sex is acceptable assuming that both parties have been tested for sexually transmitted infections and practice monogamy.

Note: Braces and jewelery should be removed prior to engaging in oral or manual stimulation of a pierced partner to avoid risk of ripping the skin.

General Intimate Piercings

Some intimate piercings are unisex. People may get them for reasons of fashion or physical stimulation, and generally, piercing devotees claim that they enhance sexual interplay. Although they are surprisingly safe and resilient to manipulation, it is worth asking a partner with a piercing to demonstrate ways in which the piercing should be manipulated.

NIPPLE PIERCINGS. Generally speaking, nipple piercings take the form of a ring. These can be licked and softly tugged, though only when sober and not under the influence of recreational drugs, to avoid accidental damage. In addition, the piercing may be circled in its hole to stimulate the areola. Should both parties have nipple piercings, care should be taken not to get them entangled.

TONGUE PIERCINGS. One of the most common intimate piercings, tongue piercing may enhance oral coitus, particularly when played over the frenulum or clitoris. In addition, a small tongue vibrator may be attached to the piercing to further intensify sensation.

Male Piercings

- Prince Albert/Reverse Prince Albert: A Prince Albert piercing goes through the frenulum and urethra, while a Reverse Prince Albert enters through the urethra and exits through a hole pierced in the top of the glans. Both allow for stimulation of the urethra by circling the piercing within the hole. If a woman has a sensitive cervix, the Prince Albert may cause discomfort during coitus.

- Shaft ampallang: This piercing penetrates the shaft of the penis horizontally at some point along its length. Again, this can give pleasure if manually toyed with, though it is best to ask the pierced partner to demonstrate. However, care should be taken during oral coitus to minimize the risk of chipped teeth or a damaged tongue or soft palate.
- Transcrotal piercing: This piercing passes through the entire scrotum from back to front or side to side. Care should be taken during testicle play to ensure that it doesn't get caught unwittingly in the teeth or hair. This is one of the most dangerous piercings to get and should only be performed by a piercing expert.
- Dydoe: A dydoe is a piercing through the ridge of the glans. This can add extra stimulation for both parties during coitus. However, there is a risk of the piercing "migrating," so the area should be checked regularly.
- Frenulum piercing: As the name suggests, a frenulum piercing goes through the frenulum, on the underside of the penis. This heightens sensitivity, particularly during oral sex, and can also enhance sexual pleasure for the female during coitus.
- Guiche piercing: This piercing is positioned through the perineum. Tantric practitioners believe this is the "root chakra," which is the sexual energy point of the body. Care should be taken during external prostate stimulation to ensure that the piercing is not pushed into the body.

Female Piercings

- Clitoral hood piercing: As the name suggests, this is a piercing of the clitoral hood, which is one of the most common female genital piercings. It is unlikely that a woman with a highly sensitive clitoris would get a clitoral hood piercing, because it increases stimulation. Indeed, some women report climax purely from the sensation of the piercing rubbing against underwear. Vibrations can intensify sensation but should be used on the lowest setting to ensure that the area is not overstimulated.
- Clitoris piercing: Clitoral piercings are relatively rare, but can be located vertically or horizontally in a woman with a large enough clitoris. Again, this massively increases sensitivity. As such, coitus may be easiest from the rear, particularly in the early stages of recovery.
- Christina piercing: A Christina piercing is located where the outer labia meet, below the pubic mound. This may be used as a form of chastity, either self-imposed or as part of a sub-dom relationship. Generally, a Christina piercing should be removed prior to sex, though leaving the piercing in place can enhance oral coitus. Anal coitus with the Christina piercing in place should only be attempted if both parties are extremely careful to minimize the risk of accidental vaginal penetration and subsequent tearing.

- Labial piercing: Similar to a Christina piercing, this piercing goes through the labia and often appears in symmetrical pairs. Again, this should be removed prior to coitus, though oral-genital contact is not prohibited.
- Fourchette piercing: The female equivalent of a male Guiche piercing, the fourchette is a labial piercing at the rear rim of the vagina. Again, this can be used to enhance Tantric sex, but care should be taken not to press the fourchette piercing inward to avoid the risk of it entering the body.
- Triangle piercing: One of the more complicated female piercings, a triangle piercing passes from side to side through the base of the clitoral hood tissue where it meets the labia, and under the clitoris. This allows stimulation of the clitoris from the rear, which may be beneficial during rear-entry coital positions.

ANALYZING AND HONING THE EFFECTIVENESS OF YOUR APPROACH

With correct study of your own genitals, you should now have a basic understanding of the appropriate stimulation that is required based on the characteristics that you have identified. In addition, you should be able to identify the ideal genital match for your body's unique traits.

To advance to the next chapter, please ensure that you have:

- Familiarized yourself with the general male and female genital structures
- Measured and categorized your genitals in terms of sensitivity and stimulation preference
- Familiarized yourself with anomalies that may be encountered in the field (extra credit for field research)
- Written an outline of the desired genital traits in a sexual partner

Once this level of comprehension has been achieved, you may progress to finding an appropriate research partner.

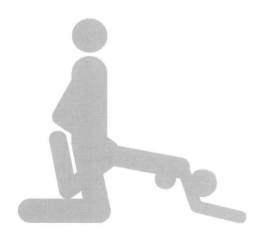

Chapter 2:

The Best Ways to Find an Appropriate Research Partner

DEVELOPING AN UNDERSTANDING OF THE OPPOSITE SEX TO ASSIST WITH MATING STRATEGIES

Now that you are equipped with a thorough understanding of both your own genitalia and that which you are likely to encounter in the field, it is time to progress to the next step: finding an appropriate research partner. The temptation to dive straight into fieldwork with the first person who comes along can be immense. However, before entering into more advanced study, it is worth identifying a study partner who offers the potential for optimal results.

ANALYZING VERBAL AND NONVERBAL COMMUNICATION TO INDICATE DESIRE

Many tomes have been written about finding a "perfect partner" based on personality and shared interests. However, this guide is concerned primarily with the sexual. Biology has a large part to play in the act of attraction, and by ensuring that these primal indicators are not ignored, the keen scholar can identify sexually compatible mates.

Whether these mates are also pleasing as potential romantic partners is something that each student must decide for him- or herself before progressing further. However, the neophyte student may be surprised at the effectiveness of paying heed to the body's primal urges.

PHEROMONES: THE INFLUENCE OF THE OLFACTORY ORGANS ON AROUSAL

Many scientists—and snake oil salesmen—have endeavored to harness the secret of pheromones, the body's natural attractant. However, as yet, there is no magical bottle of pheromones that is sure to attract a mate.

There is a very good reason for this. Pheromones act as a biological marker, attracting people who have a complementary immune system to your own. As such, there is no single pheromone that would, or should, work for everyone. Instead, your own unique pheromones will attract a mate who is the most likely to help you create healthy children—whether or not you have any desire to procreate. These pheromones will influence whether you think a fellow research partner smells or tastes right. Ignore them at your peril, as they indicate a basic biological compatibility.

Pheromones are not unique to *Homo sapiens*. Moths, sea urchins, and bees all rely on pheromones to signal their sexual desires. Indeed, such is the power of pheromones that some moths can detect a potential mate up to 10 kilometers (6.2 miles) away.

Humans excrete pheromones through the groin and armpits. Therefore, while removing armpit and pubic hair may be a cultural preference, particularly in women, it is counterintuitive, as it may reduce a female's natural chemical draw by limiting the means of pheromone distribution.

Osculation—colloquially referred to as kissing—gives both parties the opportunity to exchange pheromones through the nasal sulcus, the area of skin between the base of the nostrils and the upper lip. This explains why a kiss with the "right" person can set the nerves alight: it is literally chemistry coming into play.

One of the reasons that pheromones are so powerful is that they are processed through the vomeronasal organ (VNO) in the base of each nostril. This signal is sent directly to the hypothalamus, which is the emotional center of the brain, bypassing higher cognition circuits. As such, the "gut feeling" that someone "smells right" is little more than an unmoderated transmission of pheromones to the brain, bypassing all logic.

Although this may sound unromantic, it has formed the basis of *Homo sapiens'* mating rituals for thousands of years. And given that $12 billion is spent annually on perfumes in Europe and the United States (source: worldwatch.org), we clearly realize that smell is an essential part of mating; but again, our expenditure is counterintuitive, as we wash our natural pheromones away and replace them with unnatural—and less effective—chemical alternatives.

USING CUNNING LINGUISTICS IN MATING STRATEGIES

Although the general words that one uses are unimportant, and indeed, a UCLA study found that 93 percent of communication is nonverbal, there is something to be gained in establishing what kind of communicator you are and what kind of communicator a potential mate may be, as people tend to bond more with those who share the same communication style. In addition, sharing a preferred means of communication allows more scope for sexual compatibility.

There are four main categories of communicators: visual, auditory, kinesthetic, and auditory-digital. These can be identified as follows:

VISUAL COMMUNICATORS. The use of phrases such as "I see" and words such as "colorful," "red hot," and "bright" tends to indicate a visual person. Sexually, this person is less likely to respond to talking dirty and more likely to become aroused watching an adult film.

AUDITORY COMMUNICATORS. Auditory communicators will use phrases such as "I hear what you're saying" and "I like the sound of that." The auditory communicator will generally find dirty talk arousing and will also enjoy talking about sex. However, such types are also liable to be distracted by other noises, so music may hamper sex rather than being the "food of love."

KINESTHETIC COMMUNICATORS. Driven by touch, the kinesthetic communicator will use phrases such as "I feel" and descriptors such as "warm," "cuddly," or "touching." Driven primarily by the physical, kinesthetic communicators respond to actions rather than words. Use nonsexual touches to the arms, lower thighs, or other nonsexual regions to attract a kinesthetic communicator.

AUDITORY-DIGITAL COMMUNICATORS. Auditory-digital communicators are logic driven, and will use phrases such as "I think" or "in my experience." Sexually, an auditory-digital communicator will respond well to reading a sex manual or following detailed instructions, ideally with a statistical edge ("In my experience, oral sex is most likely to give me an orgasm").

By first identifying your own communication style, then finding a research partner who shares that style, successful congress is more likely to be achieved.

ESTABLISHING THE PARAMETERS OF PERVERSION

Establishing the specific physical and psychosexual desires that a partner has before congress is considered can limit unsuccessful sexual encounters. This is particularly important should you have any fetishes that are essential to you for pleasurable congress, or suspect that a potential mate may have hidden desires.

Clothing may give a clue as to someone's physical desires. Tattoos and piercings are common on the fetish scene, though not everyone with tattoos or piercings is a fetishist. Similarly, vintage clothing, rubber, and brightly colored hair are also abundant on the kink scene. In addition, a sexually submissive person may wear a collar to indicate his or her preference (though this can also indicate "ownership" by a dominant partner), while a dominant person may opt for biker boots or thigh boots to indicate his or her sexual status. However, many submissive and dominant people carry no overt signs of their sexuality.

Luckily, such information can be gleaned with relative ease through standard conversation, perhaps using the conversational prop of a magazine article (whether real or imagined) to distance oneself from the subject matter and thus glean a genuine reaction. For example, "Have you seen the catwalk is full of bondage clothing at the moment? What do you think about it?" Many people are nervous about sharing their sexual fetishes but become open to discussion if they realize there is no risk of negative judgment.

It is also worth paying attention to body language. Submissive partners may position themselves in such a way that they are looking up at the person they are talking to. A dominant person will take up maximum space by putting the hands on the hips or spreading the legs wide. The latter is particularly common in men.

A DOMINANT PERSON WILL TAKE UP MAXIMUM SPACE BY PUTTING THE HANDS ON THE HIPS OR SPREADING THE LEGS WIDE. THE LATTER IS PARTICULARLY COMMON IN MEN.

Although it is only during later levels of fieldwork that a person's true physical desires will become apparent, initial speculative research may help avoid an erotic mismatch. As such, it is well worth delaying coitus until a basic understanding of a potential mate's sexual preferences has been gained. The "three date rule" should allow sufficient time to gain the information you need.

SEXUAL SPECIATION: HOW EVOLUTION AFFECTS MATING SELECTION

Speciation refers to the formation of a new species as a result of physiological, anatomical, or behavioral factors that prevent previously interbreeding populations from breeding with each other. Most famously, humans speciated away from chimpanzees 4.1 million years ago—perhaps giving an indication of why humans tend to prefer less-hairy mates.

Although speciation is generally used as a term describing animal sexual behavior, there is anecdotal evidence to suggest that it may apply to *Homo sapiens'* mating rituals as well. Humans do not develop speciation to the degree that a male and a female are biologically incompatible, but certain body type pairings are more liable to lead to sexual nirvana. For example, a man with a large phallus is best paired with a woman who has an insensitive cervix and a vagina that can easily accommodate him. Going against this ideal is liable to lead to vaginal chafing and possibly related conditions such as cystitis or thrush, which will then limit opportunities for sexual pairing. Conversely, a man with a small penis is best paired with a woman who has a tight vagina or the limited friction may lead to sexual frustration and a reduction in coitus.

Although it is difficult to establish genital size in the initial stages of courting, once osculation is achieved, it is easy for the female scholar to establish the male's genital proportions because the penis will swell. Light petting can also give an indication of what to expect. Sadly, there is no outward indication of a woman's genital structure, other than the presence or absence of children in her life. Even this cannot be taken as a guarantee of a tight or loose vagina, however, as genetics and exercise can both affect the genital structure.

If you prefer a particular "type" of mate, it could be a subconscious indicator of speciation at work. Although this preference can limit your options, it may also help you identify a partner offering a higher chance of coital compatibility. More research is required into this fascinating area.

COMMUNICATING DESIRE IN THE OPTIMAL WAY

Once a suitable mate has been identified, the next task is to establish whether the attraction is mutual. Much time can be wasted pursuing a disinterested mate, so it is far more efficacious to move on to a more receptive target.

Body language offers numerous clues as to a person's level of affinity for a prospective partner. Some body language is generic. Both genders will "mirror" (copy) the posture and movements of a prospective mate whom they are attracted to. Gestures will be "open" (uncrossed, rather than crossed, arms and legs; no blockages such as a handbag or glass placed between the two parties). Nonsexual touch is frequent, with small pats to the arms or removal of fluff from someone's clothing being common. Eye contact will be more lingering than usual and blinking is more frequent. Shirt or blouse buttons may be undone, or sleeves rolled up with a grooming gesture that indicates undressing is on the subject's mind. In addition, people show attraction by licking or biting their own lips, offering a subliminal echo of what they'd like to do with the prospective mate.

Many body language signals are gender specific. If a woman is attracted to a man, she'll expose her wrists or palms to show vulnerability. She may also play with her hair, jewelery, or, at a more base level, phallic objects such as beer bottles. Women are also prone to look at a desired mate from underneath the eyelashes, showing deference to a man's masculinity. This is not a political statement, but rather a biologically driven response.

Conversely, a male who is drawn to a female will emphasize his masculinity by taking up more space, spreading his legs, or raising the volume of his voice. He may hold his head in a more upright position and stand up straighter to appear taller. Further, a male who is in the presence of a potential mate may hook his fingers into his belt loop, with his fingers pointing downward, offering a subliminal clue as to where he'd like to be touched.

Should at least three of these signals be in evidence, it is safe to assume that the potential study partner is willing. However, if only one or two signals are evident, collect further data before initiating sexual approach.

HOMO SAPIENS' MATING RITUALS

Should a polite approach be met with a rebuff, it does not always indicate guaranteed disinterest. While "no" should always be taken to mean "no" in a sexual context, the initial stages of courtship may be affected by societal conventions. Females in particular are inclined to "play hard to get" in an effort to appear chaste.

An entire subculture of self-titled PUAs (pick-up artists) or "seducers" has evolved over the past decade to share tips on how to break through these barriers. Some of the advice shared is morally spurious, but there are several astute, psychologically based methods that may prove useful to males with a poor grasp of seduction techniques.

LOOK POPULAR. A male who is surrounded by a crowd of people will be believed to have a higher social status than one standing alone. This perceived status will help attract a female mate.

INITIATE CONTACT RAPIDLY. It is recommended that an interested male approach a potential female target within three seconds of seeing her. Hesitation allows time for your cognitive processes to induce a fear response, which can hamper easy conversation. Assert your sexual interest rapidly, though subtly, in the first five minutes, to avoid being perceived as a potential friend rather than lover.

BE DISMISSIVE. Although it may seem counterintuitive, the adage "treat them mean and keep them keen" is sadly effective. This does not mean being openly insulting, but instead using gentle teasing to provoke a desire in the female target to prove you wrong.

Attractive women are used to being complimented, but if that compliment comes with a sting in the tail, it creates "cognitive dissonance" in which a woman's brain tries to process why she's been rejected, and she subconsciously tries to win your approval. Use this technique sparingly, however, or you will simply be perceived as rude.

Use neuro-linguistic programming. Commonly known as NLP, neuro-linguistic programming is used by therapists to help get through blockages on a subconscious level. It relies on linguistic ambiguity—using phrases or words that sound alike but differ in meaning, such as blow and below—to plant subliminal sexual thoughts in a woman's head.

Should all of these tactics fail, the keen scholar is best advised to seek a new study partner, as the attraction is purely one-way.

A PERSON WHO APPEARS TO HAVE THIN LIPS MAY HAVE MEDIUM-SIZE OR EVEN FULL LIPS AFTER AN EXTENDED BOUT OF KISSING, THOUGH THIS CHANGE IS ONLY TEMPORARY.

SEDUCTION OF A POTENTIAL MATE: THE ROLE OF OSCULATION

Once a potential mate has been identified and courted, it is time to enter the physical realm. After initial courtship, it is generally expected that osculation will occur. The point at which the lips meet is the moment at which you can first establish whether predicted compatibility has a grounding in reality.

Should a kiss prove disappointing, and not the product of poor technique, this is a solid indicator that further research is unlikely to yield beneficial results. Whereas technique can be corrected, a lack of chemistry suggests a biological incompatibility.

ANATOMICAL STRUCTURE OF THE MOUTH AND LIPS

It is worth considering oral structure prior to oscula-tion, as the shape of the lips, mouth, and teeth can all affect the compatibility of the kiss. Osculation is often more effective between people with similarly sized mouths and lips; otherwise, the partner with the smaller mouth may find the experience involves excessive levels of saliva around the lips.

In addition, partners with larger mouths may feel that they are taking a dominant role, as their lips will surround those of a smaller-mouthed lover during kissing. While this may not be a problem if the person with the larger mouth is content in a dominant role, it is preferable to be able to assume both dominant and submissive roles during the course of a relationship.

As with genital structure, first ascertain your own characteristics before assessing those of the potential field partner.

Size and Shape of the Mouth

SMALL MOUTH. Although small mouths are generally deemed to be less sexually appealing than larger mouths with fuller lips, this physical attribute should not hamper sexual activity. However, a woman with a small mouth may wish to avoid men with large members, as oral coitus may be uncomfortable.

If a small-mouthed woman has a large vagina, and thus requires a partner who is well endowed, different oral sex techniques can be used to ensure her partner is satisfied, and manual stimulation may form more of a part of oral coitus than is standard. Ensure that lots of lubrication is used, as this will help create the sensation of oral penetration when teamed with a pulsating hand.

Conversely, a male with a small mouth may find extended cunnilingus tricky, particularly if paired with a woman who has a large clitoris, as it can limit the array of techniques that can be used and may necessitate repeated extensions of the tongue. (The muscles of the tongue can be developed by eating fromage blanc, yogurt, ice cream, or other types of dessert using the tongue alone. This is recommended as a solo practice because it may look risible to observers.)

However, do bear in mind that small lips can be deceptive. During osculation, the lips swell in the same way that the genitals swell during arousal. As such, a person who appears to have thin lips may have medium-size or even full lips after an extended bout of kissing, though this change is only temporary.

MEDIUM-SIZE MOUTH. Although women are deemed most attractive if they have full lips, research has found that a medium-size mouth is more attractive than a feminine full mouth on a man, according to professor Michael Cunningham, University of Louisville, Kentucky. Cunningham heads the Social Communications Laboratory, where he and his students investigate social and evolution-ary processes in romantic attraction and repulsion, making him a name that scholars should pay particular attention to.

A medium-size mouth should be acceptable for most forms of coitus, unless a female with a medium mouth couples with a man who has an exceptionally large penis, in which case oral coitus may be limited. As with a small mouth, this is easily dealt with by using manual and oral coitus in tandem.

SHOULD YOU BE IN POSSESSION OF A PARTICULARLY LARGE TONGUE, IT IS BEST USED IN MODERATION DURING SOUL KISSING TO AVOID STIFLING A PARTNER.

LARGE MOUTH AND LIPS. Often deemed the most sexually appealing type of mouth, full lips convey warmth and receptivity, a finding confirmed in Cunningham's research. In addition, by pursing the lips, a woman sends out signals that she is sexually open to advances. As such, many women try to emphasize the size of their lips using lipstick, gloss, and possibly even surgery.

Large lips offer a pillowy sensation to the person who is being kissed, and they imply arousal because they are naturally swollen. However, large mouths will, by their nature, contain more saliva, which may make the kiss wetter than standard unless the experience is being shared by two large-mouthed people. This aside, there is no sexual activity that is limited by having large lips.

Oral Anomalies Encountered in the Field

FULLNESS UNDER CUPID'S BOW. Research by Dr. Stuart Brody of the University of West Scotland has found that women who have a prominent tubercle of the upper lip, the area just underneath the Cupid's bow, are more prone to climax through vaginal penetration. However, this is only the case if it is natural, and sceptics have argued that this could simply be because women with full lips are deemed more attractive and thus may have higher self-esteem that feeds into the enjoyment of coitus. Regardless, a sexually inexperienced male scholar may choose to use this identifier to increase his chances of inducing climax in a partner.

PROTRUDING OR CROSSED TEETH. From a practical point of view, protruding teeth may limit oral coitus, particularly if a woman has a particularly

sensitive clitoris or a man has a particularly large phallus. If corrective treatment is not an option, it is particularly important to sheath the teeth with the lips or use a device such as the Blowguard dental shield to protect a mate from damage.

BRACES. The use of braces in adults is becoming increasingly common. These limit osculation if a potential mate has a tongue stud or other oral piercing. Should both parties wear braces, proceed only with extreme caution.

Similarly, penetrative fellatio is not recommended. However, much pleasure can be given using a combination of manual stimulation and licking around the area. Similarly, males with braces should ensure that they use the tip of the tongue to stimulate a partner orally, rather than pressing the mouth into the genital region.

LONG TONGUE. Although a long tongue can prove beneficial during oral coitus, it is best avoided by small-mouthed individuals, as osculation may be spatially challenged.

OSCULATORY OPTIONS EXPLORED
Having established that a partner has suitably compatible lips, there are myriad techniques that can be explored. Some techniques are more suited to particular lip combinations than others. These are detailed below.

THE ESKIMO KISS. This is a romantic rather than sexual kiss, which is best employed during early courtship stages, prior to the first kiss, and as a means of conveying affection later in a relationship. It entails rubbing the tip of your nose against a lover's nose.

This can be sexualized by exchanging breath with a lover as you rub noses together; Tantric practitioners believe that sharing breath can lead to heightened sexual pleasure and intimate connection.

Suitable for: all mouth pairings

TANTRIC BREATH EXCHANGE. Sharing breath at a deeper level can produce surprisingly effective results. Gaze into a lover's eyes with your lips a few millimeters apart. First breathe in your lover's breath, then exhale into your lover's mouth. Continue this until you are both breathing easily in the same rhythm. However, stop if either of you becomes light-headed, as it may lead to blackouts. Teaming Tantric breathing with gentle caresses to the torso, back, and buttocks offers a sensual and caring way to enjoy each other, which is as suitable to the early stages of a courtship as to a long-term relationship.

Suitable for: all mouth pairings

SOUL KISSING. Often considered to be the most sexually charged type of kiss, soul kissing entails letting your tongue explore a lover's tongue and mouth and vice versa. This is best started slowly, with limited tongue penetration until the lips start to swell.

Excessive saliva should be wiped away discreetly unless both parties prefer a wet kiss. This can be done easily by moving your attentions to a mate's neck, kissing it until the oral region is no longer covered in excessive saliva, then returning to the lips.

Should you be in possession of a particularly large tongue, it is best used in moderation during soul kissing to avoid stifling a partner.

Suitable for: small/small, small/medium, medium/medium, medium/large, and large/large pairings

SUCTION. While suction may be incorporated into osculation to enhance the experience, it is best to focus attention on the lips rather than the tongue, particularly if using extreme suction, as otherwise it is possible to break the frenulum that attaches the tongue to the base of the mouth. However, mild suction will enhance most kisses if used sparingly.

Suitable for: small/small, small/medium, medium/medium, medium/large, and large/large pairings

As with all forms of sexual activity, osculation should evolve as a relationship progresses. Applying a generic technique is purely a starting point from which more tailored techniques can be developed.

ANALYZING AND HONING THE EFFECTIVENESS OF YOUR APPROACH

After reading this chapter, you should have a thorough comprehension of the biological factors that will predispose a potentially sexually satisfying encounter.

To advance to the next chapter, please ensure that you have:

- Understood the role of pheromones in sexual attraction
- Identified a study partner's linguistic sexual preference indicators
- Gained a basic understanding of verbal and nonverbal ways to indicate desire in *Homo sapiens'* mating rituals
- Identified your own mouth shape
- Familiarized yourself with anomalies that may be encountered in the field (extra credit for field research)
- Gained an understanding of appropriate osculation techniques

Once this level of comprehension has been achieved, you may progress to understanding manual coitus. Practical demonstrations should only be sought once your research partner is keen to advance his or her own studies.

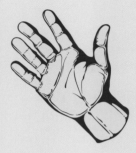

Chapter 3:

A Hands-on Approach to Mating Rituals

GAINING AN AWARENESS OF MANUAL-GENITAL CONGRESS TECHNIQUES

Manual stimulation tends to be more common in the initial stages of a relationship, before the two parties have progressed to coitus. It allows for initial exploration of the body without the same degree of intimacy as mating. This stage of study is particularly important because it allows you to fully assess the physical scope of a potential mate, and thus identify the likelihood of coital compatibility.

Before commencing intimate manual exploration, it is expected that you will proceed through milder levels of physical touch. This is not only a matter of etiquette, but also allows the student to assess a partner's preferred degrees of physical intensity.

A DIGITAL WORLD

The human hand is more complex than comparable organs in any other animal; it contains twenty-seven bones and opposable thumbs that between them allow for infinite variations of movement. As such, the hands are able to provide myriad forms of stimulation, from a sensual caress to a passionate grip.

While many people overlook hand care, ensuring that the nails are trimmed and adequately manicured to avoid hangnails and rough edges is a basic part of coital etiquette. Should the sexual scholar undertake a blue-collar profession in which the hands become callused, rough spots should either be buffed away with a pumice or, if calluses are desirable to protect against pain during manual labor, latex gloves should be worn during intimate stimulation to avoid scratching the delicate genital tissue.

Further, the hands should be washed prior to any form of intimate stimulation to decrease risk of infection.

INITIAL MANUAL APPROACHES

When first approaching a new partner, it is appropriate to progress at a leisurely place (see *Tits First, I'm No Whore! A Sexual Approach Analysis*, by Dr. Cherri Pye). This is not only to ascribe to societal norms, but also to allow arousal to be built in a steady way. The skin is the largest erogenous zone of the body, containing thousands of nerve endings, and neglecting to stimulate it prior to congress shows a rushed and naive approach to coitus.

As a general rule, touch should start at the mild end of the spectrum and only progress to more vigorous stimulation as intimacy deepens (see Physical Intensity Chart in this chapter). Simply holding hands with a potential mate can be highly sexually charged. Allowing the fingers to play between each other, altering the grip from tender to tightly grasped, and letting the fingernails delicately trace the back of your lover's hand can all signal sexual desire while being perfectly acceptable displays of public affection.

Stroking the inside of the wrist can be highly arousing, as it displays trust and intimacy. In addition, certain areas of the body are more responsive to touch, despite having a normal distribution of nerve endings. These include the inner arms, neck, sides of the torso, backs of the knees, and armpits. This is because the skin is thinner in these areas, and they are also less likely to be desensitized through friction from clothes. Stroking any of these areas is therefore liable to provoke a strong response.

Some people may find these zones too ticklish to be pleasurably stimulated, particularly in the case of the armpits. However, once you have progressed beyond hand holding, gently trailing a hand down the neck or sides of the body during osculation will generally add sensuality to the act.

Limit early physical approaches to stroking and caressing. Spending a significant amount of time engaging in nongenital foreplay will help build anticipation and deepen subsequent arousal.

Initial stroking should take place over clothing, with hands gradually slipping under clothes, buttons slowly being undone, and bra straps being pushed off. A gradually revealed body offers significantly more temptation than a rapid strip.

TICKLING CAN BE USED TO SPEED THE THROES OF PASSION, AS LAUGHTER HELPS PARTNERS BOND. HOWEVER, THIS SHOULD BE USED SPARINGLY BECAUSE MANY PEOPLE BECOME RAPIDLY IRRITATED BY THE ACT.

Tickling can be used to speed the throes of passion, as laughter helps partners bond. However, this should be used sparingly because many people become rapidly irritated by the act.

With the progression of intimacy, further types of touch may be incorporated. Cupping the buttocks during osculation or the breasts during neck kissing, indicates desire while still maintaining a degree of decorum. As passion heightens, squeezing and gripping the back, buttocks, thighs, or breasts can demonstrate desire while also triggering feelings of arousal in a mate.

MASSAGE: A PLEASURABLE APPROACH TO SEDUCTION

Often used as a precursor to coitus by the sexual sophisticate, massage offers a two-pronged benefit. First, it allows thorough exploration of the body's erogenous zones. Second, it helps relax a mate. Stress is one of the major causes of low libido. Thus, helping a mate relax prior to congress is liable to reap rewards.

There are two key strokes used in massage: petrissage (kneading) and effleurage (stroking). By varying the two, the sexual scholar can optimize the effectiveness of the massage, helping relax and arouse a partner in equal measure.

Start with long, smooth effleurage strokes of the body to establish whether there are any areas of tension. These are easily identified because they feel both tighter and more knotted than relaxed muscles do.

Once the entire body has been explored with a gently roving hand, return to the problem areas that you have identified. Ease tension with light circular motions, only increasing pressure at a mate's behest. Use petrissage to relax any extreme areas of tension, but only after the area has been sufficiently relaxed through effleurage. Massage oil or lubricant is essential to ensure that the skin does not suffer friction burns. Similarly, ensure that the room is warm and there is a blanket or towel at hand, because the body cools during relaxation, which may lead to discomfort for the person being massaged.

Avoid touching the spine because doing so can be dangerous. Instead, focus attention on the shoulder blades, along the sides of the spine, the lower back, and the buttocks. Should your hands get tired, use the elbows to press into the larger muscled areas, gently using the weight of your own body to administer pressure. Always ensure the skin is kept lubricated, as this will enhance sensuality as well as comfort.

Once a mate is suitably relaxed, you may opt to progress to more direct intimate contact, whether manually, orally, or coitally. Ensure the hands are washed before touching a lover's genitals or the lubricant may cause condoms to break during coitus.

Alternatively, you may choose to explore further methods of manual stimulation to extend anticipation and build arousal further.

STIMULATION OF THE SECONDARY EROGENOUS ZONES

Prior to initiating genital stimulation, it is wise to explore the secondary pleasure centers to ensure that your approach will be willingly accepted.

Nipple stimulation in both the female and the male causes the area to swell with blood, in much the same way as the genitals become engorged. However, the stiffening of the nipple is no indication as to sensations of arousal, in either the male or the female—it is merely a physical response that may or may not be pleasurable. Using exploratory touch combined with clear communication should help keen scholars establish whether they are following the right path.

Skillful Removal of the Brassiere

No skillful student should balk when confronted with a brassiere. Instead, it should be kept in place until the female is pushing her breasts into the student's hand or vehemently requesting that she be further stimulated in the mammary region. At this point, it should be swiftly dispatched with a single hand. This is a simple procedure that has nonetheless flummoxed many students for many years.

The initial approach should be softly exploratory to establish whether the bra fastens at the front or back. If it is the former, investigate the kind of clasp more closely under the guise of nuzzling the breast.

If it is a hook-and-eye closure, simply unhook the top of it between finger and thumb, then push the other side of the fastening upward and over. If it is a snap fastening, bring the two sides of the clasp together using your finger and thumb.

If it is a back-fastening bra, simply put your thumb underneath the bra and a finger or two on the band fastening, then push the two sides together.

Once the breasts are revealed, allow the woman to remove the bra herself. If she does not initiate this but seems happy for you to continue your ministrations, there is no need to remove the brassiere yourself. You now have full access to the breasts, so it is no longer an impediment to your caress.

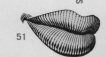

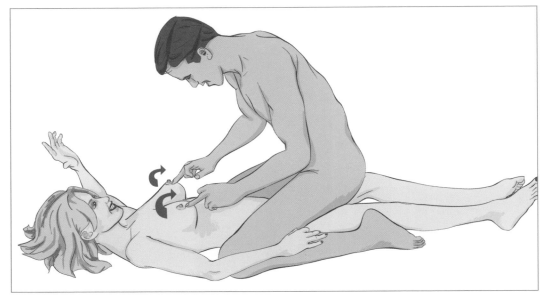

Figure 1: Focusing on the sensitive underside of the breasts in ever decreasing circles is likely to offer an erotic tease and deliver a pleasurable response.

Anecdotal stories abound referring to males "trying to tune in a radio" when attempting to toy with the nipples. This approach is not recommended. Initiating breast caresses prior to approaching the nipple is liable to garner a more receptive response. The underside of the breasts and the cleavage are frequently ignored during breast play, despite the relative sensitivity of the skin. Focusing on these areas before progressing inward in ever decreasing circles is likely to deliver a more erotic tease.

Once the focus moves to the nipples, trace your fingers lightly around the areola and pay close attention to the response. If the nipples appear to be sensitive, maintain delicate stimulation. If they appear to require further stimulation, light squeezing and pinching may prove effective. However, be gentle: overenthusiastic nipple play can be extremely painful.

Although female nipple stimulation is generally depicted as a standard form of foreplay, the dedicated male student should be aware that the nipples are not necessarily the optimal erogenous zone for a woman. Indeed, the neck, shoulders, and inner thighs are often reported to be more responsive areas when women are questioned about their preferred erogenous zones.

Conversely, while female nipple stimulation is commonly accepted as a standard part of advanced courtship, the male nipples are often neglected. While this may not be an issue to many men, a proportion of males find that there is pleasure to be gained from this form of foreplay. As such, the female student should ensure that she explores this nerve-rich area in a similar method to that detailed earlier, before progressing to more intimate parts.

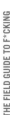

ANECDOTAL STORIES ABOUND REFERRING TO MALES "TRYING TO TUNE IN A RADIO" WHEN ATTEMPTING TO TOY WITH THE NIPPLES. THIS APPROACH IS NOT RECOMMENDED.

ADDITIONAL NONGENITAL METHODS OF MANUAL PLEASURING

While popular opinion tends to assume that congress has evolved and modern sexual practices are more sophisticated than those practiced in the past, in reality, texts as ancient as the Kama Sutra outline numerous types of caressing that may still be considered extreme, such as scratching, slapping, and hair pulling. Although modern depictions of these acts in adult videos often focus on threatening and degrading behavior, the skilled lover can utilize all of these forms of touch in a way that enhances pleasure without objectifying a partner in a negative way.

SCRATCHING AND PINCHING. The Kama Sutra categorizes the art of scratching with great levels of detail, such as marking the body with half-moons, a circle, or a "tiger's claw," utilizing the nails to demonstrate love or passion, or leaving a lover with a reminder of oneself during a period of separation. It also recommends suitable times to engage in scratching: on the first visit, when setting out on a journey, upon return from the journey, when an angry lover is reconciled, and when a woman is intoxicated.

This information may seem shocking to the contemporary scholar and, indeed, it is most definitely inadvisable to use a state of intoxication as an excuse to enter into any sexual encounter. Similarly, scratching on initial contact may be considered more than a little forward. However, once a relationship has been established, there is certainly truth in the concept that marking a lover in such an intimate way may help trigger positive memories during a period of absence.

Whereas the Kama Sutra recommends marking a partner in public places such as the décolletage, modern culture tends to frown upon such sexual markings, identifying public scratches (and indeed, love bites) as being an indicator of immaturity or low morals. Instead, scratches should be employed in more private places, such as the inner thighs or buttocks, ensuring the only person who knows the markings are there is the person who has been intimately marked. The genitals should not be scratched because this may lead to infection.

Pinching is another form of touch that can combine pain and pleasure. However, it should be used in moderation, and focused on fleshy areas such as the buttocks or breasts unless more thorough pinching is specifically requested by a mate. In extreme cases, you may wish to employ clothespins or nipple clamps for pinching, should this be to a partner's taste.

SLAPPING. While slapping a partner without consent is never acceptable, incorporating loving slaps into sex play can increase passion. It suggests an animal nature that can be appealing on a primal level. Play fights can form an entertaining method of foreplay, as long as both parties are fully consenting and no actual harm is administered.

Spanking, in particular, is a popular fetish and has solid scientific benefits. When the body is slapped, it produces painkilling endorphins that can provide a natural high. This is most effective if slaps start gently and gradually increase in intensity once the brain's endorphins start to flow through the body. For safety, spanking should be limited to the buttocks and thighs, and under no circumstance should you strike a lover's lower back because you may inadvertently hit the kidneys, which can cause serious harm.

Should spanking be deemed too extreme, you may wish to proceed at a milder level, with a gentle slap to the buttocks as a teasing gesture (or during coitus, once you have progressed to that level).

Conversely, should you wish to entertain more niche practices, slapping the face can be arousing to a submissive partner and used as part of a sub-dom fantasy, though again, only with prior consent and mutual desire. Care should be taken to ensure that you don't inadvertently hit the ear, as this may cause the eardrum to pop, and rings should be removed prior to slapping to avoid accidental nicks and bruises.

PHYSICAL INTENSITY CHART

Stroking **1**

Caressing **2**

Tickling **3**

Cupping **4**

Squeezing **5**

Gripping **6**

Pinching **7**

Pulling **8**

Scratching **9**

Slapping **10**

Note: Should a partner wish to transcend this scale, students should ensure their mate indicates the maximum physical intensity parameters that he or she is comfortable working within.

HAIR PULLING. Hair pulling may be deemed too extreme for many people, but there is no reason for it to be as crass or violent as it is presented in contemporary adult films. Washing a partner's hair can be enhanced by gently tugging on the hair while lathering it, as this helps relax the muscles of the scalp. Gripping a partner's hair during fellatio or cunnilingus can help indicate your desires, and tugging the head back by the hair during a passionate kiss can also demonstrate arousal.

At a milder level, stroking the hair at the nape of the neck before gently pulling it to tilt a lover's head backward and initiate a kiss combines both passion and sensuality in equal measure. And should you wish to explore a more animal experience together, pulling the hair back during doggy-style sex may appeal.

LEAVING BASE CAMP: MANUAL MANIPULATION OF THE PRIMARY EROGENOUS ZONES

After adequate osculation and nongenital touch, the logical progression is genital manipulation. There are numerous manual techniques that can be employed in the genital region to thoroughly stimulate every centimeter, whether as a form of precoital arousal generation or as a sole means to invoke climax in a partner.

Manual congress is not simply a case of manipulating your partner's genitals using a certain technique. It's about playing with the mind as much as the body. It allows you to give pleasure in the ultimately selfless way, devoting yourself to ensuring that your mate receives as much sexual pleasure as possible without experiencing any direct stimulation yourself (though, obviously, dual stimulation is possible in numerous ways).

By paying as much attention to the details of manual stimulation as to those of coitus, the sexual scholar will achieve top marks. Both hands should be used, and almost all other body parts should be considered to add extra stimulation.

MANUAL MANIPULATION OF THE FEMALE GENITAL REGION

As you learned in chapter 1, the female genital region comprises six main areas: the mons, clitoris, vagina, cervix, G-spot, and A-zone. Further, some women enjoy manual manipulation of the anal region. While the latter will be covered later in this chapter, there is no reason that a digitally dexterous student should not be able to stimulate all of these areas simultaneously if required.

Many people make the mistake of using a sole hand, when expert manipulation should involve both hands. One hand can thus be used to part a lover's labia or cup her mons and clitoris, while the other focuses on penetration of one or both intimate orifices. Having a basic toy chest (see Essential Toolbox: Ensuring Adequate Provisions for Optimal Congress in this chapter) will extend the scope further.

Manual stimulation allows you to use all of the knowledge acquired in chapter 1, tailoring your sexual techniques to the genitalia of your study partner. These techniques should be considered as options to choose from and combine based on the exact specification of your partner, rather than as an absolute rule. They are a tool kit from which to pick and choose. Your ministrations, however, should take into account the anatomical structure of your study partner's genitalia, as outlined in the following sections.

Size of the Clitoris

SMALL CLITORIS. Digitally manipulating a small clitoris can be problematic, as it may be hard to locate. The easiest way to approach the small clitoris is to take a lubricated finger and slide it from the vaginal opening upward toward the pubic mound, feeling carefully for an area that swells when caressed. Take a slow and steady approach, making small circles with the fingers to ensure that every inch is covered.

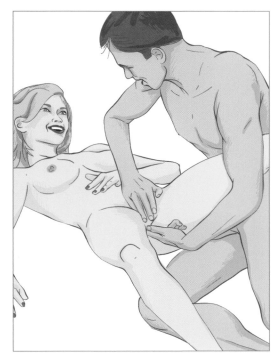

Figure 2: Cupping the pubic mound with the fingers facing downward provides indirect stimulation to a small clitoris. You can use the fingers of your other hand to penetrate your partner's vagina or anus or both, depending on her preference.

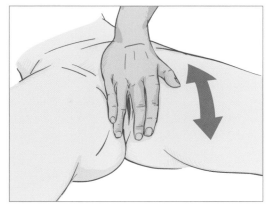

Figure 3: Keen scholars can move their fingers into a V shape, extended downward over the labia and clitoris, and then rock them up and down to stimulate a medium clitoris.

Once found, rub slowly to encourage the clitoris to swell. You may wish to use a bullet vibrator to speed the process. Penetrating the vagina with the middle finger, while the thumb is extended upward will help stimulate the clitoris.

If the clitoris proves too elusive, opt for pubic mound stimulation instead, cupping the mound with the fingers facing downward toward the vaginal opening, as this will give indirect stimulation to the clitoris, even if you are unable to feel any changes. Use the fingers of the other hand to penetrate the vagina, anus, or both depending on the preference of your study partner.

MEDIUM CLITORIS. The medium-size clitoris can be pleasured using various techniques. Try spreading your fingers into a V shape, with the fingers extending downward over the labia and the clitoris in the point at which the fingers meet. Then rock your fingers up and down. You can use the fingers of the other hand to penetrate one or both orifices.

Alternatively, you can strum lubricated fingers from left to right or up and down across the clitoris. It is always worth trying both options and paying attention to your lover's response, as different women prefer different directional motions (see *Don't Bring Your Ex into the Bedroom: An Analysis of Technique Adaptivity*, by Dr. Alec Change).

Some women respond well to light squeezing of the clitoris. You can also tap it with your fingers, squeeze it between the labia majora, or stroke the clitoris with the thumb and one finger of the same hand while you penetrate the vagina and/or anus with one or more fingers of the other hand.

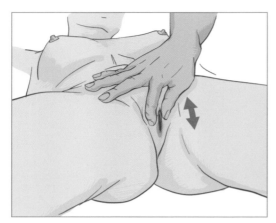

Figure 4: You can treat the large clitoris as a miniature phallus and try masturbating the shaft between two fingers.

LARGE CLITORIS. A large clitoris offers the most scope in terms of technique. In addition to the techniques detailed for the smaller clitoris, you can treat the large clitoris as a miniature phallus. It is best not to refer to this as a tactic to your partner, however, as, much like men, no woman wants to hear that she has a small penis. Instead, simply use this knowledge to inform your sexual technique.

Try masturbating the shaft of the clitoris between two fingers, possibly using fingers of the other hand to penetrate the vagina, anus, or both. Rub a lubricated heel of the hand over the mons and clitoris in large circles, squeeze the clitoris between thumb and finger, or cup the mons and clitoris from behind, with your lover on all fours, using the fingers of the other hand for penetration. Resist the urge to wink at yourself in the mirror should you find yourself in this fortunate position, as it may offend your study partner.

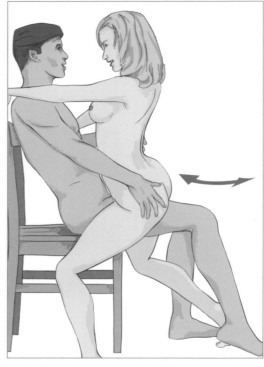

Figure 5: Some women find grinding themselves against their partner's thigh offers sufficient stimulation should their clitoris prove too sensitive to direct stimulation.

Sensitivity of the Clitoris

EXTREMELY SENSITIVE CLITORIS. Some women may find the clitoris too sensitive to be touched at all. If so, rub the pubic mound with the heel of your hand, or apply indirect stimulation instead. A woman with a sensitive clitoris may respond well to straddling your thigh and controlling the level of friction herself by grinding against you. Alternatively, if her clitoris is too sensitive for any stimulation at all, opt for rear entry using your fingers on her labia and for penetration only. While the clitoris is generally the key to female orgasm, you won't unleash anything pleasurable by trying to force the lock.

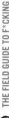

WHILE THE CLITORIS IS GENERALLY THE KEY TO FEMALE ORGASM, YOU WON'T UNLEASH ANYTHING PLEASURABLE BY TRYING TO FORCE THE LOCK.

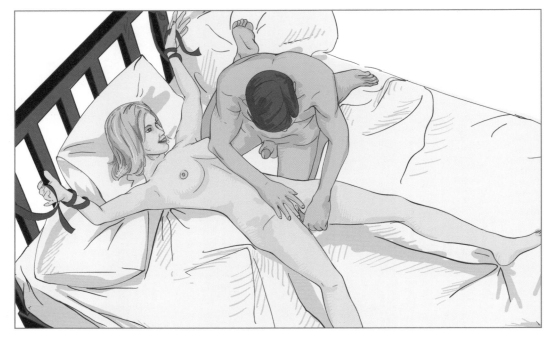

Figure 6: Try using a vibrator on a mildly insensitive clitoris to increase stimulation levels. You can couple this with some form of fantasy role-play, such as appealing to her dominant or submissive tendencies.

SENSITIVE CLITORIS. A sensitive clitoris should only ever be approached with a well-lubricated hand (and ideally, all manual play should be preceded by a liberal coating of lubricant, regardless of a woman's clitoral sensitivity level). Again, it is best to avoid direct stimulation, as it is liable to be painful. Instead, push the labia together gently, to apply indirect stimulation to the clitoris. Again, stimulating the pubic mound is likely to bring pleasure to your lover without causing any pain. Do not assume that your manliness gives you the power to make her clitoris crave your touch despite its innate sensitivity. Female nerve endings have no role to play in appeasing your ego, and attempting to overrule them will result in a reduction in coital opportunity.

RESPONSIVE CLITORIS. A responsive clitoris can be pleasured in numerous ways. It can be lightly tapped with the pad of the finger, stroked along its length or girth with a lubricated fingertip, and gently squeezed or teased indirectly by cupping the entire pubic mound. You can approach the responsive clitoris with a bullet vibrator, though always start on the gentlest setting unless you know a more rigorous form of stimulation is desired. And you can combine penetration with clitoral stimulation using a two-pronged toy or a finger and bullet combination, or up the ante to triple stimulation using a three-pronged toy or both hands and a butt plug or vibrator. Do bear in mind that this approach may be deemed a little forward for the first date.

It is advisable to shop for the requisite toys together to avoid any psychological trauma caused by contemplation about the sex toys' heritage.

Essential Toolbox: Ensuring Adequate Provisions for Optimal Congress

Should further stimulation be required, or single-handed manipulation be preferred to leave the other hand free for self-stimulation, there are numerous devices that can be purchased to aid your endeavors. An ideal sexual toolbox (colloquially referred to as a "toy chest") should contain:

- A multispeed bullet vibrator
- Silicone and/or water-based lubricant
- A phallic dildo, ideally Perspex or crystal
- A vibrator with clitoral stimulator (or dual prongs for triple stimulation of the clitoris, vagina, and anus)
- 6 meters (2 yards) of bondage rope
- Cuffs (whether silk, metal, leather, or Velcro)
- Vibrating cock ring
- Butt plug

These tools allow for maximum provision of variation but need not cost any more than a reasonable dinner for two, despite providing years' worth of pleasure.

In addition, prophylactics should be included for use during congress unless both parties have been tested for sexually transmitted infections and pregnancy prevention is in place. These should include delay condoms, warming condoms, extra-safe condoms, flavored condoms, and standard condoms of an appropriate size.

Condom sizes are listed on the backs of the packets. Using the penile measurement technique outlined in Measuring Criteria for Optimal Genital Sizing, it is thus possible to choose a condom of ideal size. Anecdotal evidence suggests that many males who had previously reported issues with prophylactics found all negative side effects to vanish when issued a condom of appropriate size (see article, *If It's Uncomfortable, You're Too Big: Tight Condom Syndrome Explained*).

MILDLY INSENSITIVE CLITORIS. When approaching a mildly insensitive clitoris, it is wise to engage the mind as well as the body. Some form of dirty talk or fantasy role-playing may help increase the arousal of the woman. If she has submissive tendencies, tying her legs apart or cuffing her wrists (with informed consent) may also increase stimulation levels.

Vibrators come into their own when confronted with an insensitive clitoris. Try using one hand to squeeze the clitoris while the other plays a bullet vibrator along its length. Or, use a multiple-pronged toy for stimulation of the G-spot, vagina, cervix, labia, and other genital erogenous zones.

Nipple stimulation may also help provide extra sensual arousal to speed climax. The woman with an insensitive clitoris offers an adventure playground of exploration: just ensure that you follow any safety warnings to the letter.

EXTREMELY INSENSITIVE CLITORIS. An extremely insensitive clitoris is likely to become considerably more responsive if the clitoral hood is retracted, either by using a finger lubricated by saliva (lubricant may be too slippery and encourage the clitoris to become elusive to your touch) or by pressing the heel of the hand into the pubic mound. This then exposes the clitoral tip, which can be stimulated using the fingers or a vibrating device of any description.

Again, bringing fantasy into the fold may be of benefit. In extreme cases, you may opt for using mild clitoral clamps or a clothespin. However, in opting for these methods it is wise to remember that the pain increases upon releasing the clamp. As such, you should never take someone to her maximum pain threshold when clamping her, but instead take her almost to the edge.

Anal, G-spot, or breast stimulation, or possibly all three, may also be required to bring a woman with an extremely insensitive clitoris to climax. While this may sound like excessive work, the scholar should relish the opportunity to explore such fertile ground.

Note: Regardless of the sensitivity of a woman's clitoris, it is worth remembering that the area becomes much more highly sensitized immediately after climax. Direct contact may become painful and, though it may be tempting, continuing to tease a woman's clitoris after climax is more likely to lead to reticence when future sexual approaches are made than it is to spur her on to greater heights. If you wish to continue sexual activity after a woman's climax, give her time to recover—ideally by urging her to pleasure you in some way. This has two benefits: no pain for the woman and a greater amount of foreplay for the male.

Size of the Labia

SMALL LABIA. Small labia may be hard to pleasure during manual stimulation, as the scope is rather limited. That said, you can squeeze the entire labial area together while stimulating the clitoris. Running a vibrator along the labia will encourage them to swell, which may then allow for more direct methods of stimulation.

MEDIUM LABIA. Medium labia can easily be pulled apart, gently, to allow deeper penetration of the fingers during manual stimulation. They can also be stroked and squeezed, and if the woman has pubic hair, she may find it pleasurable if you lightly tug downward, as this will cause the clitoral hood to move over the sensitive clitoral tip.

LARGE LABIA. Large labia offer themselves up to the greatest array of manual stimulation techniques. They can be parted or squeezed, stroked, or masturbated between finger and thumb. This will indirectly stimulate the clitoris and can be used as a delay technique, should you wish to have an extended foreplay session without leading the female to climax, to heighten the eventual release.

Size of the Vagina

SMALL VAGINA. Although it is often cited that the vagina can stretch to accommodate a baby's head, the fact that drugs are frequently used to facilitate this process is generally omitted. As such, when approaching a small vagina, it is best to chart a careful course. Do not penetrate the vagina until there is sufficient natural lubrication to easily insert a digit. Although lubricants can be used to assist, without natural arousal it is unlikely that the cervix will tilt backward, thus increasing the risk that deep penetration will be painful.

Use clitoral stimulation throughout to ensure an adequate flow of lubrication and remember that, if anal toys are used, this will further tighten the vagina.

Should you wish to involve a toy, choose a slender model. Some women with small vaginas are simply tight, while others have a sensitive cervix that limits depth of penetration. Choose the length of toy accordingly. Should the shaft of a rabbit-style toy be too thick for a partner with a small vagina, opt for customizing your own version using her toy of preference with a vibrating cock ring around the base to add clitoral stimulation. This approach can also be used to modify the phallus.

MEDIUM VAGINA. A medium-size vagina may require the use of more than one digit for stimulation. However, fingers should always be added one at a time to ensure that there is no uncomfortable stretching. In addition, do bear in mind that flexing the fingers changes the shape of the knuckles, which may then cause discomfort.

Toys may be used to increase stimulation. As a general recommendation, choose toys with your partner rather than separately, as this will help ensure that the right item is procured. Turning up with a maxi-vibro dong when one's partner would prefer a clitoral butterfly can lead to relationship conflict.

LARGE VAGINA. Should a woman's vagina be of sufficient size that stimulation with the fingers alone is not enough, you may wish to consider vaginal fisting. While this is an extremely niche act that has been represented in an often unpleasant way in adult films, if done in a gentle and caring fashion, it can offer deep and thrilling stimulation. As with all sex acts, it should only ever be entered into with full, informed consent.

When introducing the hand into the vagina, the fingers should not be formed into a fist, despite the name of the act. Instead, the fingers should be drawn as closely together as possible, with particular care given to minimizing the breadth of the knuckles. Fisting should start with standard digital penetration using one finger, and additional fingers should only be added once sufficient vaginal lubrication is produced. Clitoral stimulation will increase speed of lubrication.

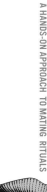

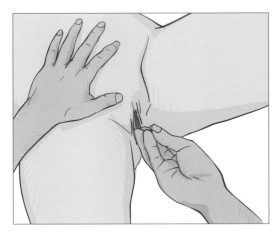

Figure 7: Consider fisting for large vaginas that need additional stimulation. Begin by drawing the fingers close together and inserting them one at a time into the vagina, going slowly so that it gets used to the sensation and can become suitably aroused.

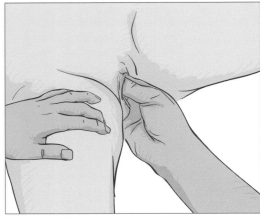

Figure 8: Next, cover the hand in lubrication and slowly insert the entire hand into the vagina, with the thumb pressed into the palm to minimize the size of the fist. Allow the woman to set the pace throughout to ensure her comfort.

Once the vagina is suitably aroused to accept a fist, cover the entire hand in lubricant to ease its ingress. Push the fingers into the vagina, taking it extremely slowly, and pause at the first knuckle of the fingers to allow the vagina to accommodate the hand. Once the vagina is suitably relaxed, continue to push forward or, alternatively, ask your partner to push her hips toward your hand. This has the advantage of ensuring that the pace is ideal. Softly twist the hand from side to side once the second finger knuckles are reached to further ease entry.

Once the finger knuckles are inside, again pause to allow the vagina to adapt to the hand, only pushing forward at your partner's behest. Ensure the thumb is tucked into the palm of the hand to minimize the size of the fist, and again, twist when attempting to slide the hand into the vagina beyond the thumb knuckle. If there is discomfort at any point, stop immediately and slowly withdraw the hand. However, do remember that the thumb joint is at the widest point of the hand, and pressing forward will allow the vagina to relax around the comparatively smaller wrist.

Once the hand is inside the vagina, it is wise to allow the woman to set the pace. She may wish to grasp the wrist of the hand to control the depth of penetration, pace of movement, and eventual egress of the hand. This is most easily done during the throes of orgasm, rather than afterward, as the body's natural convulsions will serve to assist.

Obviously, there is a complex interrelation to consider when entering into manual (and indeed, any) sex play. A woman may have a sensitive clitoris but a large vagina that requires deep penetration. If so, the student is advised to use common sense to draw on the appropriate techniques for each aspect of genital structure (in this instance, by penetrating deeply from behind, to avoid stimulating the clitoris). Ensuring a solid communication flow throughout manual stimulation will help avoid any unsuitable techniques.

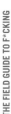

Deep Stimulation

Manual stimulation is ideal for a woman who enjoys deep penetration, as she can be pleasured in multiple ways, regardless of the male's phallic dimensions. Stimulation of the G-spot, A-zone, and cervix all require similar positioning and, as such, will be covered in this section.

The optimal position for deep penetration with the fingers is from the rear. Thus, the woman should kneel on all fours or bend over a bed or the arm of a sofa. Should this position be undesirable for the woman (for example, because she is insecure about the size of her buttocks), a similar effect can be gained if the woman raises her legs in the air. The higher the legs are raised, the deeper penetration will be, meaning that resting the ankles on the ears offers the maximum benefit. Should this position be uncomfortable to maintain for a period of time, you may wish to use pillows underneath the buttocks and hips.

Bondage can also be of assistance for deep stimulation, as it allows the keen student to hold the female in a position that provides maximum access to the vagina et al. while still leaving both hands free for exploration. Simply ask the female to raise her legs to fully expose the genital region, then tie her ankles to the bedpost (obviously, this should only be done with informed consent). Alternatively, the woman can simply hold her ankles above her head.

Speedy penetration with the fingers tends to offer deeper penetration. However, this also carries the greatest risk of scratches, so take extra care to ensure that your fingernails are short and buffed, or wear latex gloves to cover your nails.

Alternatively, toys may be used, and are available in multiple lengths and girths. You may also wish to consider vaginal fisting (see the earlier section on Large Vaginas) if a woman craves extremely deep penetration. This has the advantage that it is almost impossible to avoid stimulating the G-spot and A-zone.

Conversely, if a female finds deep penetration uncomfortable, focus on clitoral stimulation and external play. Allow the woman to guide your hand when indulging in any penetrative practices, as this allows her to clearly indicate the depth that she is comfortable with. Toys should be used with care, as it is easy to get carried away given the comparative lack of feedback gained from a toy rather than your own fingers.

MANUAL MANIPULATION OF THE MALE GENITAL REGION

As with women, it is important to consider all parts of the male genital structure when instigating manual stimulation. Many people focus purely on masturbating the shaft and rubbing the glans, ignoring the intricacies of the foreskin, coronal ridge, frenulum, and meatus. While there is still pleasure to be offered using such an unsophisticated approach, the entire experience will benefit by paying attention to detail.

Anal stimulation is more of a taboo in the heterosexual male than in the homosexual male, but there is potential for great pleasure through stimulation of the prostate gland. As with female sexual coitus of the anal variety, this will be dealt with in detail later in this chapter.

Using both hands is as essential with the male as it is with the female. One hand may be used to masturbate the shaft while the other (well-lubricated) hand can circle around the glans. Alternatively, you may wish to consider cupping or tugging the testicles with one hand while the other moves the foreskin up and down over the glans; or simply use both hands simultaneously to masturbate the shaft. Again, referring back to the toy chest may allow for further exploration and stimulation.

These techniques should be considered as a seduction arsenal from which to select manual coitus options based on the exact specifications of your partner, rather than as techniques to be followed to the letter.

Size of the Penis

The size of a penis has a great impact on the manner in which one should approach manual stimulation. As a general rule, males like to feel as if they are well endowed. As such, the role of the hands is to maximize this perception: the objective is to ensure that the females' hands seem as small as possible to make the phallus appear comparatively larger.

For example, holding the penis at the base leaves the maximum amount of phallus visible, suggesting that the male is too large to fit into his partner's womanly hands. This act provides a subliminal ego boost, making the male feel more "manly." While there is no research into this area to date, and as such any extrapolation should be treated with due skepticism, it would not be unfeasible to believe this positive reinforcement could increase a man's testosterone level and subsequent sex drive (see *You're So Big!: Phallic Praise and Its Role in Self-Actualization*, by Dr. Simon Z. Matters).

Larger members will require a dual-handed approach on the shaft and glans alone, turning toys into a necessity for additional stimulation. The toolbox detailed above contains all that you need to approach a phallus of any size.

SMALL PENIS. A small phallus will generally exert less strain on the wrists, making extended pleasuring easier. Assuming the male has a positive response to testicular stimulation, using one hand to tug on the testicles while the other masturbates the shaft will serve the dual purpose of providing thrilling stimulation and increasing the apparent size of the penis.

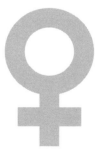

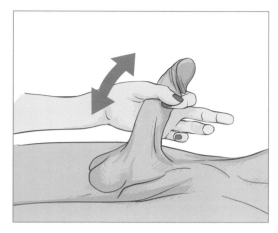

Figure 9: Rather than using your whole hand to stimulate a small phallus, form your thumb and index finger into an O and slide it over the glans and up and down the shaft.

Rather than using the whole hand, form your thumb and index finger into an O shape, as if indicating that it is okay the male study partner has a small member, and use this to slide over the glans and up and down the shaft. Again, this will make the phallus appear larger.

Speeding movements is a matter of ease, and the remaining fingers of the hand can be played over the testicles to add extra stimulation. This leaves the other hand free to explore the neck, nipples, testicles, or anus. Do not attempt the latter without prior consultation. Uninvited rectal probing tends to be poorly received in both male and female subjects.

Lubrication, Lubrication, Lubrication

One essential, regardless of the phallus you are confronted with, is to use lubricant. Without lubricant, extended periods of penile stimulation will cause chafing, which can then lead to loss of desire for coitus. Though a saltwater bath will help speed recovery and ensure the penis is fit for coitus, it is preferable to avoid this issue in the first place.

Water-based lubricants will dry more rapidly than silicone-based lubricants. However, they are generally cheaper and can be reactivated by spraying with water (keep a spray bottle filled with clean tap water or mineral water next to the bed). Silicone lubricants are more slippery (though the latest water-based lubricants now come very close). This makes them ideal for anal play. However, if you have wooden floors, exercise extreme caution, as any spillages are both exceptionally hard to clean up and prone to making the floor highly slippery.

UNINVITED RECTAL PROBING TENDS TO BE POORLY RECEIVED IN BOTH MALE AND FEMALE SUBJECTS.

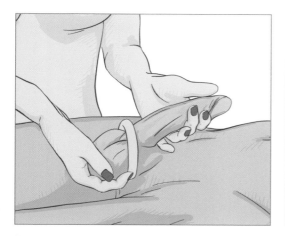

Figure 10: Sliding a cock ring onto a fully erect penis will prevent blood from flowing out of the penis, ensuring it stays firm. Cock rings can be positioned at the base of the shaft or behind the balls.

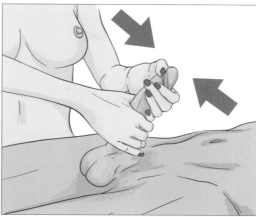

Figure 11: Use both hands when it comes to a large penis, encasing the shaft and the head of the penis.

MEDIUM PENIS. A medium penis will appear bigger if the pubic hair is removed. In addition, once erection has been fully achieved, slide a cock ring, ideally with at least one vibrating attachment, onto the penis. This will prevent blood from leaving the penis, ensuring that it stays in an optimal state of firmness.

The shaft should be stimulated using one hand, while the other hand caresses the glans or explores the testicles and anus. Should the cock ring have two bullet attachments, one to stimulate the clitoris and another to stimulate the perineum, press the fingers of one hand lightly into the perineum stimulator as the other masturbates the shaft and glans. This provides male G-spot stimulation without requiring entry into the anus (see *Slowly Does It: An Anal Sex Primer*, by Dr. A. R. Stockter).

LARGE PENIS. A large penis will generally require both hands to encase both the shaft and the head of the penis in full. Squeezing both hands together simultaneously along the entire length of the penis, or rippling the hands to emulate the rippling of a vagina, is likely to garner a positive response. Indeed, one of the keys to successful male stimulation is emulating a vagina at all times: warm, wet, and tight teasing is liable to garner a positive response regardless of the method used to produce the sensation.

Female scholars without experience of male ingenuity in pursuit of a vaginal experience should read *Portnoy's Complaint* by Philip Roth to better familiarize themselves with masturbatory methods considered acceptable by the average male. Any psychological trauma experienced as a result of this knowledge is the scholar's own liability.

Should a single-handed approach be preferred to leave the other hand free for exploration of the neck, nipples, testicles, and anus, or for self-stimulation, a larger vibrating cock ring may be employed to stimulate the base of the penis. Alternatively, a butt plug or nipple clamps may be used to stimulate other areas of the body.

Sensitivity of the Penis

Although penis size has an impact on hand positioning, technique will equally be dictated by the sensitivity of the penis. Multiple forms of stimulation are generally recommended, but should the male study partner have an extremely sensitive penis, this level of stimulation may speed ejaculation to unacceptable levels. Conversely, a male who has a desensitized penis may find it near impossible to ejaculate without extreme levels of stimulation. Clearly, these factors need to be taken into consideration alongside those concerning phallic size. A penis, as a man, should not be judged by appearance alone.

EXTREMELY SENSITIVE PENIS. An extremely sensitive penis may ejaculate with such speed that manual-genital congress can only be used as a sex act in its own right, rather than as a form of foreplay. A delay lubricant may help minimize this risk.

However, rapid ejaculation need not be an issue as long as it is understood by both parties. Many men who suffer from premature ejaculation are able to maintain further erections after initial climax and find that subsequent sexual activity induces climax at a much slower rate. As such, ejaculation during manual stimulation is little more than the first course in an extended sexual meal.

SENSITIVE PENIS. A sensitive penis should be able to take firmer handling without immediate ejaculation. Approach gently, initially stroking the penis and testicles before progressing to lightly grasping the penis. Move slowly and change technique regularly to slow climax. Alternate stimulation of the penis with caresses to the testicles or possibly anal penetration. Alternatively, a delay lubricant may help prolong foreplay. Some practitioners recommend squeezing behind the glans of the penis firmly as a way to ward off ejaculation. This is not to be recommended without prior warning as it may otherwise kill the mood rather more fatally than scholars may wish.

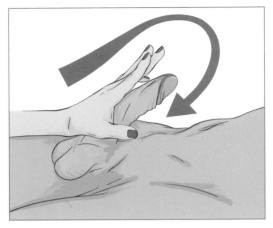

Figure 12: Swirling your palm up the shaft of the penis, around the head, and then back down the shaft tends to garner a positive reaction from a responsive penis. Use lubricant on your palm to keep things moving smoothly.

RESPONSIVE PENIS. A responsive penis can be stimulated in a variety of ways. As with all manual-genital stimulation, lubricant is recommended. However, the formulation you opt for is a matter of personal preference. Many companies sell sample sizes, allowing you to choose a lubricant that is right for you.

Masturbating the shaft while swirling a well-lubricated palm around the head of the penis may take a little practice but tends to garner a positive response. Try different grips, from a loose, rapidly moving hand to a firmer gripping and pulsing palm. Should guidance be required, it is highly likely the male study partner has honed his expertise in the area and will be fully equipped to demonstrate his preferred masturbatory methods.

MILDLY INSENSITIVE PENIS. If a man has issues with penile sensation, multiple levels of stimulation may well be required. Consider incorporating testicle or anal play into manual-genital congress, and remember that men tend to be visually stimulated.

SHOULD GUIDANCE BE REQUIRED, IT IS HIGHLY LIKELY THE MALE STUDY PARTNER HAS HONED HIS EXPERTISE IN THE AREA AND WILL BE FULLY EQUIPPED TO DEMONSTRATE HIS PREFERRED MASTURBATORY METHODS.

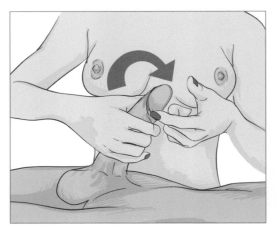

Figure 13: Holding the shaft of an insensitive penis while lightly circling the coronal ridge with the finger of your other hand can induce pleasurable sensations.

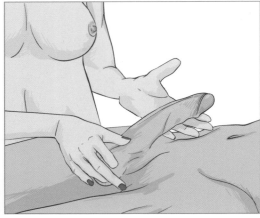

Figure 14: Focusing attention on the perineum may also have a positive effect without directly stimulating the testicles.

As such, wearing sexy lingerie or masturbating yourself while manually pleasuring the male may help speed climax. This act will also be appreciated by males in general.

Adult films are another option to consider, if you do not have any ethical objections. There are many feminist pornography producers in today's world, and adult films are now available depicting consensual, loving sex in addition to more hard-core acts.

EXTREMELY INSENSITIVE PENIS. A male who suffers from an extremely insensitive penis is advised to show his lover the manner in which he indulges in self-pleasure to best assist her endeavors. Stimulation of multiple areas, such as the nipples, inner thighs, testicles, and anus, may also be beneficial. The meatus may be more sensitive than the rest of the penis, as it is less exposed to friction than the rest of the phallus. As such, gently circling it with a well-lubricated finger, though not penetrating it, may induce pleasurable sensations.

Sensitivity of the Testicles

It is easy to ignore the testicles during manual coitus, or worse, accidentally knock them, which can cause bruising. However, with appropriate caresses, testicular stimulation can be a wonderful addition to sex play.

SENSITIVE TESTICLES. A man with sensitive testicles may object to manual stimulation entirely. If you do approach them, opt for skimming the fingers over the hair of the testicles lightly, rather than cupping or squeezing the testicles. Focusing attention on the perineum may also have a positive effect without directly stimulating the testicles. If in doubt, don't.

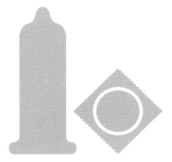

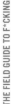

Cut and Uncut

The foreskin can be a useful part of the anatomy in manual-genital congress, as it both lubricates the glans and provides possibilities for sex play. However, there is no reason that a circumcised male cannot enjoy equal sexual pleasure if the right techniques are employed.

CIRCUMCISED. As previously mentioned, lubricant is essential rather than desirable when dealing with a circumcised male. Applying lubricant in creative ways can help make this part of the sex act. Try pouring lubricant over the breasts, then using them to apply the lubricant (in an act colloquially referred to as a "tit fuck" or a "Russian"). Alternatively, lubricate the penis orally, adding extra lubricant once manual stimulation commences, because saliva alone will not be enough.

The coronal ridge may be either highly sensitized or utterly lacking in sensation in the circumcised male. Explore gently with the soft pad of a finger, and increase pressure on demand. The frenulum should be approached in a similar way.

UNCIRCUMCISED. Do not neglect the foreskin of an uncircumcised male during manual stimulation. It should be used as a guide as to the effectiveness of the techniques being employed. Gently hold the head of the penis underneath the foreskin and slowly slide it up and down the head of the penis. Alternatively, start with your hand at the base of the penis, and slowly move it up the shaft, "collecting" the foreskin on the upward stroke and gently easing it over the head of the penis.

As the male becomes more aroused, his foreskin will retract, much as the clitoral hood retracts during female arousal. If the glans is not sufficiently lubricated by this time, add extra lubricant to minimize the risk of chafing.

RESPONSIVE TESTICLES. Try cupping and tugging on the testicles while masturbating the shaft. The testicles can also offer a seductive way in which to initiate manual congress, as stroking the testicles is intimate but less demanding than grabbing the penis directly. Listen to your partner's language, both verbal and nonverbal, to assess the appropriate next step. A positive response is likely to be visually clear.

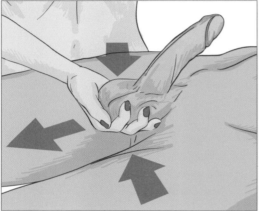

Figure 15: As well as stroking and cupping testicles, tugging them may draw a pleasurable response.

INSENSITIVE TESTICLES. A male with insensitive testicles may require squeezing of the area in addition to cupping and tugging, but do ensure that you are still gentle. In addition, pressing relatively firmly on the perineum may help increase sensation. Reassure your study partner that there will be no unexpected anal play because perineum stimulation can lead to tension in the male.

PERIPHERAL ENGAGEMENT IN ALTERNATIVE PRACTICES

Although the majority of people dislike pain, there is a substantial minority that enjoys the complex sensation of combining pleasure with pain. This is no new perversion, but rather an age-old part of human sexuality.

The Marquis de Sade gave his name to the practice of sadism, due to his penchant for whipping servant wenches and committing many acts that even the most broad-minded student might balk at. Conversely, masochism—gaining sexual pleasure from experiencing pain or degradation—derived its name from Leopold von Sacher-Masoch, whose book *Venus in Furs* explored themes of male pain and humiliation. More recently, fashion designers such as Jean Paul Gaultier have drawn inspiration from BDSM (bondage, domination, sadism, and masochism) fetish wear, and barely a day goes by without a popular music entertainer making allusions to spanking, bondage, or "being a bad girl."

In short, the keen scholar should have a thorough understanding of basic BDSM acts from little more than access to popular culture. However, it is worth understanding a bit more about common techniques before commencing such play.

CLAMPING. Clamps may be used on the nipples, labia, or scrotum while administering manual-genital stimulation. These vary in complexity from the simple clothespin to multiple-gauged clamps offering an array of degrees of pressure. Because this is an extreme sex act, it is essential that you have a safe word in play prior to commencing clamping. In addition, do not forget that clamps are most painful when removed, as the blood rushes back into the area. Thus, pressure should only be applied to near-maximum levels rather than pushing a partner to the furthest reaches of his or her pain threshold.

ANAL PENETRATION. Many people are satisfied with manual-genital contact alone, but some prefer the addition of anal stimulation—or, indeed, find anal stimulation more pleasurable. Although it is still considered a taboo act by many, there is no reason that the anal region should be neglected during sex play as long as appropriate care is taken.

Hygiene is scrupulously important, for matters of both taste and infection. Ensure that the partner who is being anally stimulated has bathed or showered thoroughly prior to commencing the act. The fingernails of the penetrating partner should be cut short and buffed smooth. Alternatively, latex gloves can cover long fingernails and also offer a guard should you have any cuts on your fingers or simply feel squeamish. It is possible to contract *E. coli* and other diseases through unsafe anal play, so latex gloves are a good protective measure. If you opt to practice manual stimulation of the anus without gloves, ensure that you wash your hands thoroughly before any other genital contact, and keep the fingers well away from the oral cavity of either partner.

Lubricant is also essential. Ideally, one should opt for a silicone-based lubricant, because it is more slippery. However, a water-based lubricant will suffice. Under no circumstance should you use petroleum jelly or an oil-based lubricant because this can cause irritation of the delicate anal tissue.

Anal penetration should always start slowly, as the delicate anal tissue can easily tear, which may cause painful fissures. Circle a lubricated finger around the anus until the muscle relaxes. Continue to circle the finger around the anus, drawing ever nearer, until the fingertip rests against the entrance.

Slip just the tip of the finger inside the anus and allow the muscle to relax further before progressing. This may take several minutes, but rushing will simply cause the muscle to tighten and require commencing external stimulation once more.

As the sphincter relaxes, push the finger slowly forward, or ask your partner to push back against your finger. Alternatively, let your partner guide your movements, whether verbally or by holding on to your hand as you stimulate the anus. There should be constant communication during anal stimulation. This should not be an issue and, indeed, may be of benefit to your sex life (see An Anal Analysis). Add lubricant at regular intervals, to ensure that there is no uncomfortable friction.

When stimulating a male anally, press gently against the back wall of the anus as you penetrate it, until you find an area that feels like a walnut and swells when stimulated. This is the prostate gland, also referred to as the male G-spot. Its sensitivity varies from individual to individual. Some males find anal penetration a psychological challenge (in which case it is worth remembering that anal stimulation is no indication of sexual preference) or physically uncomfortable (though there is no need for this to be the case as long as the guidelines here are followed). Others find that stimulation of the prostate gland can lead to climax without any phallic play. At the very least, every male should explore his prostate gland, as it can be a pathway to intense orgasms.

When stimulating a female, it is advisable to team anal stimulation with clitoral or vaginal stimulation, as there is no specific erogenous zone inside the female anus. However, the area is still rich in nerve endings, and female orgasm is more common if anal stimulation is incorporated into sex (see An Anal Analysis). Do ensure that any finger or toy that has stimulated the anus is thoroughly cleaned before entering the vagina or it can lead to infection.

The anus does not stretch as much as the vagina does. As such, the novice student is advised to start with a single finger, and perhaps progress to a small butt plug. This is likely to be easier to accept than multiple fingers, as butt plugs are designed in the optimum shape for anal penetration. Once you are used to anal penetration, you may choose to move on to penetration with multiple fingers or larger toys, but this is certainly not something to be rushed into. Further, bear in mind that a toy offers less feedback than fingers do, so it may be advisable to ask the partner who is being anally penetrated to insert the butt plug, and only start manipulating it once it has been comfortably accommodated.

Because of the construction of the anus, thrusting in and out may be more painful for the receiver than gently moving the finger or toy from side to side or up and down inside the anus. This is because the sphincter tightens every time the penetrating item is fully removed. Once high levels of arousal have

An Anal Analysis

Recent research into sexual behavior found that 94 percent of women who had had anal sex during the sexual encounter that immediately preceded the study had attained climax, compared to 81 percent who had had oral sex and 65 percent who had had penetrative sex.

Interpreting this data raises interesting questions. Is anal sex the most effective form of female stimulation? Although that interpretation would no doubt garner a positive response in many male scholars, an equally likely hypothesis is that couples who practice anal sex are less likely to feel guilty about sex, as they are engaging in an act that is still deemed taboo in many places, and feeling able to transgress against social norms in this way suggests a lack of sexual inhibition.

Further, couples practicing anal sex need to communicate more clearly to ensure the act is not painful. This communication then feeds into their sex life as a whole, benefiting every aspect of sex.

In addition, couples practicing anal sex were likely to have entered into oral and vaginal coitus during the same sexual interlude. A commonsense analysis would suggest that stimulation of multiple zones provides a more satisfying sexual encounter for the female. However, dedicated students may wish to read the results in full, available online, to extrapolate their own findings from the data given. (Source: *National Survey of Sexual Health and Behavior 2011*, Center for Sexual Health Promotion, Indiana University, sexualhealth.indiana.edu/publications.html.)

been achieved, the sphincter may relax enough to allow more vigorous movements, but this should only be attempted after thorough communication with a partner.

Anal penetration may form part of foreplay or may lead to climax in its own right. Indeed, there is no reason that both options need not be the case. However, it is worth bearing in mind that, after climax, the anal region may become highly sensitized. As such, it is worth removing any fingers or toys as soon as climax has been reached to ensure that your partner does not suffer any pain.

Now wash your hands.

SIGNS OF AROUSAL AND HOW THEY VARY

Now that you have progressed to more intimate exploration of a partner, it is important to be aware of signs of arousal in addition to basic body language. Although these vary massively from individual to individual, common traits include:

- Speeding of the breath
- Flushing of the skin, particularly the face and chest
- Tightening of the thigh muscles
- Pointing of the toes
- Increase in blood flow to the clitoris or penis
- Increased quantity of sexual juices

In addition, there are vocalizations of myriad types that can be emitted, ranging from groans and squeals to cursing and blasphemy. This should provide a clear guide as to the efficacy of your stimulation. If a partner remains silent, this does not necessarily mean that he or she is lacking in arousal. Some people are quiet during sex because of feelings of self-consciousness, while others find that vocalizations distract the focus from climax. However, if your partner is the silent type, it is particularly important that you pay attention to his or her body's responses.

Finally, it is worth being aware of some of the anomalies that may be encountered upon climax. It is possible that you may encounter a partner who laughs at the point of climax, possibly because of the intense relaxation that orgasm can induce. A partner may also cry, not out of sadness but as a result of the chemicals released at the point of orgasm (if genuinely upsetting crying is induced, it is worth the tearful party seeking counseling, because there may be unresolved issues relating to sex). Anecdotal reports also suggest that hiccupping after sex is not uncommon. Flatulence may also occur as a result of the sudden relaxation of the muscles. This is to be discouraged and, if it happens on a regular basis, an immediate exodus to the lavatory after climax is to be recommended, in an attempt to protect your partner from the odious gas.

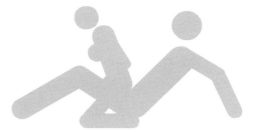

ANALYZING AND HONING THE EFFECTIVENESS OF YOUR APPROACH

After reading this chapter, you should have a thorough comprehension of the ways in which the hands can be used for skillful manipulation of the primary and secondary erogenous zones.

To advance to the next chapter, please ensure that you have:

- Understood the correct way to instigate initial manual approaches
- Attained clear comprehension of the different types of manual stimulation
- Learned how to remove different types of brassiere with ease (extra credit for field research)
- Learned how to stimulate the primary and secondary erogenous zones in a partner of either gender
- Gained comprehension of the ways in which scratching, slapping, pinching, and hair pulling may be incorporated into sex play with a consenting partner
- Familiarized yourself with the Physical Intensity Chart
- Created a sexual toolbox
- Developed an understanding of the importance of lubrication
- Gained an understanding of alternative sexual practices, including clamping, anal penetration, and vaginal fisting
- Learned about the various ways in which arousal may be shown
- Assessed the likelihood of advancing beyond manual-genital stimulation to oral-genital contact or congress

Once this level of comprehension has been achieved, you may progress to studying oral-genital congress, ideally incorporating the lessons learned about manual-genital congress to combine the two arts, where appropriate. Practical demonstrations should only be sought once your research partner is keen to advance his or her studies.

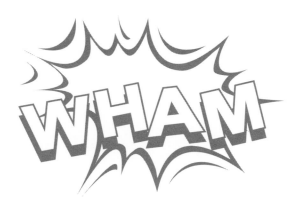

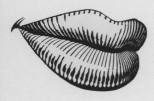

Chapter 4:

Understanding Oral-Genital Congress

ORAL STIMULATION OF THE GENITAL REGION

The act of oral-genital congress has long attracted controversy. Although it is undoubtedly one of life's greatest erotic delights and is often cited as the easiest way to help the female of the species achieve climax, there is still a stigma about it. Indeed, many American states have labeled the act as criminal over the past century, while others have deemed it acceptable only within a marital relationship (see *The Fringe Benefits of Marriage*, by Dr. Peter Proud).

Contrary to misguided opinion, the act of using the mouth to manipulate the genital region offers no hazards to one's health or psyche, assuming standard levels of hygiene and health care are followed.

Although many texts focus on the general techniques required to orally manipulate a penis or vagina to provoke an orgasmic response, the sophisticated student should first ensure a basic biological compatibility. The shape and size of the upper labial region, commonly referred to as the mouth, must be taken into consideration before commencing oral copulation to ensure optimal results.

AN ORAL ANALYSIS

There is no ideal mouth formation for oral sex, simply an ideal match. An incorrect oral-genital pairing may lead to chafing of the vagina or penis, and can also provide a choke hazard during fellatio, particularly with a novice male who fails to adequately understand the mechanism of the gag reflex while inflicting excessive thrusting on his mate.

The oral region can be broken down into four main constituents, all of which need to be considered before commencing oral-genital contact.

THE LIPS

The male heterosexual is commonly attracted to women with oversized lips, often referred to colloquially as a "cocksucker mouth." The fullness not only provides the penis with a stimulating sensation upon entry and a key visual arousal tool during the act, but also implies fertility on a subconscious level. The brain is seemingly unable to comprehend the low likelihood of impregnation via oral stimulation, instead focusing on the perceived youth of the female fellatrix, which provides a powerful, primal urge to ejaculate.

In addition, the female lips are often cited as offering a "genital echo," planting images of the lower labia in the mind of the heterosexual male. As such, both lipstick and lip gloss provide an enticing signal: the former, indicating that the lips are swollen with blood, as with arousal; the latter, as an indicator of wetness.

Male lips are also important in the act of cunnilingus. Full lips provide a gentle pillow with which to stimulate the clitoris. Thin lips can be a barrier to attraction, indicating an uneasy proximity of the clitoris to the potential mate's teeth. Chewing and sucking thin lips will help increase the fullness and thus counter this negative signal. However, this should be performed in private and kept to a minimum to ensure that the lips do not become chapped.

Chapped lips provide both visual and sensory barriers to effective oral-genital contact. Dry skin should be removed by brushing the lips with a soft toothbrush, after which petroleum jelly or lip balm should be applied to speed healing. Licking the lips may act as a visual attractant, but it should be used sparingly as a technique to limit risk of chapping.

THE MOUTH

The naive sexual explorer may ignore the mouth entirely when contemplating oral congress. However, to do so is an amateur's mistake. In the act of cunnilingus, levels of saliva produced in the mouth can make a significant difference to overall sensation. During fellatio, both the size of the mouth and the level of gag reflex need to be taken into account, in addition to salivary response.

Should saliva levels be less than ideal, the problem is easily rectified through hydration. Although the oft-touted figure that 75 percent of Americans are dehydrated has been shown to have little scientific basis, it is true that dehydration will lead to lower levels of saliva production. Further, imbibing alcohol can lead to "dry mouth," which may have a negative effect on cunnilingus and fellatio techniques.

It is also worth taking into account the size of a potential mate's mouth. A well-endowed man may find a partner with a small mouth or tight jaw is incapable of providing full oral-genital satisfaction. Conversely, a man with full lips and a large mouth may struggle when faced with an extremely small clitoris. A woman with an extremely sensitive clitoris may find cunnilingus most enjoyable when administered by a man with full lips; a man who is lacking in penile sensitivity may experience greater pleasure from a woman with firm, strong lips.

Finally, the gag reflex should be taken into consideration during the act of fellatio. Although it is possible to train the gag reflex (see *Cucumber Deep Throating: A Primer*, by Dr. Sally Swallow), this takes time and is not something to be attempted during oral-genital congress unless it is mutually agreed upon.

Other contraindicated acts with an initiate mate include holding the back of a partner's head during fellatio, thrusting deeply during the initial stages of the act, and ejaculating without warning. While these acts are frequently depicted in films of an adult nature, they should only be explored with a willing and gag-reflex-trained partner.

A well-endowed man may find that oral-genital congress is limited with a partner who lacks gag reflex control. Conversely, a man with a small member may find his perfect match in a woman who has yet to enter into gag reflex training, as she may well be able to satisfy him without engaging in further study.

The Pain-Phobic Alternative to Tongue Piercing

Should tongue piercing be a step too far in one's quest for sexual nirvana, an alternative is available in the form of the Tongue Joy vibrator, which attaches to the tongue via means of an elastic band. Preparing oneself to use the Tongue Joy is an inelegant process, requiring extending the tongue to its maximum length. Saliva levels may also be vastly increased during the process, leading to excessive drooling. As such, it is advised that the Tongue Joy be put in position when students are in a solitary state, only to be revealed to a partner through the act of oral-genital congress.

THE TONGUE

The tongue has an essential role to play in oral-genital congress. According to Guinness World Records, the longest tongue in the world is 9.8 cm (3.87 inches) long, and a male who is blessed with a long tongue may find it ideal for "tongue fucking," offering a pleasurable alternative to penile penetration.

Although this length of tongue is clearly ideal for penetrative cunnilingus, a long tongue is by no means essential for effective oral stimulation. Flickering a small tongue over the clitoris or glans can be just as pleasurable as allowing a long tongue to sweep over the entire area. And for the purposes of fellatio, a long tongue may hinder progress, blocking the path of the penis into the throat.

In addition, it is worth considering the effect of tongue piercings, particularly if lack of sensitivity is an issue during oral-genital congress. Although this is still very much a minority-supported body modification, advocates claim that the additional stimulation offered by the ball of the piercing can enhance the sensation of oral sex, making a pierced partner ideal for people with lack of genital sensation. It is also now possible to buy tongue vibrators that attach to a piercings base.

THE TEETH

It is worth considering a potential mate's tooth formation before progressing to oral congress. Should a prospective partner have an overly crowded mouth, it may limit pleasure.

Male students in particular may experience dentaphobia—the fear of teeth taking a more central role than is proper during oral-genital congress. As such, it is essential to ensure that the teeth are adequately covered while administering fellatio. The most common way to do this is to use the lips to cover the teeth before penile penetration of the oral cavity commences. However, should this prove problematic, the Blowguard is a tool created by a dentist to minimize the risk of accidental biting. This simple shield fits over the teeth, covering them with soft silicone. The additional vibrating bullet provides extra intensity to oral sex acts.

Conversely, a woman with a particularly sensitive clitoris may experience discomfort should her partner have an overbite with crossed-over teeth, as this may increase proximity to the sharp biting edges of the teeth. Should this be the case, using tongue extension rather than close mouth-to-genital contact may help minimize risk.

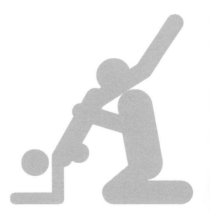

Understanding and Overcoming Objections to Oral-Genital Congress

The genitals are still a taboo subject in many cultures. As such, the concept of oral-genital contact is still deemed shocking by some. Common—and apocryphal—objections to the act include claims that it is unhygienic, is immoral, and may cause infertility. However, there is no reason that oral-genital congress should be unpleasant for either party, assuming that the genitals are suitably clean.

The sophisticated lover may also consider removing the pubic hair via shaving or depilatory methods to minimize the risk of choking a mate with an errant hair. Brushing the pubic hair prior to oral sex to remove any loose hairs can serve as a low-maintenance middle ground.

Should a partner take issue with the act of oral-genital congress, it is worth exploring the motivation behind the fear. A thoughtless prior lover may have created psychological issues through inappropriate behavior, such as holding the head during oral sex, or neglecting personal hygiene levels. These fears must be tackled in a sensitive manner.

Coping mechanisms may include sharing a shower together before commencing oral-genital exploration, using flavored lubricants to mask the natural taste of the body, or agreeing to indulge in oral sex only up to the point of extreme arousal, changing to manual or coital stimulation before climax. Any mate who expects to indulge in nonreciprocal oral-genital contact should be promptly disabused of this notion unless there is an extremely valid reason for such selfish behavior.

IT IS FAR BETTER
TO UNDERSTIMULATE A PARTNER,
MAKING HER BEG FOR ADDITIONAL
STIMULATION, THAN TO KILL THE MOOD
WITH OVERENTHUSIASTIC AND PAIN-
INDUCING TECHNIQUES (SEE *SHE
WON'T TELL YOU, BUT SHE WILL TELL
HER FRIENDS: FEMALE RESPONSE TO
POOR MALE SEXUAL TECHNIQUE,*
BY DR. HONOR BOUND).

In addition to these considerations, oral hygiene can be an indicator of general cleanliness levels. As such, if a desired mate has stained, chopped, or rotten teeth, it may be worth contemplating whether it is worth taking the risk of entering into an intimate situation. Should the risk be deemed worthy of the reward, introducing the concept of foreplay in the bath or shower prior to removing clothes may help ensure the experience is not limited by hygiene factors. Offer your study partner mouthwash after using it yourself to psychologically coerce said partner into using it, too. Alternatively, mint tea or even schnapps may help, should you really insist on pursuing a malodorous mate.

THE BASICS OF CUNNILINGUS

The optimal cunnilingus technique is not simply about pushing the face into the genitals and letting the tongue explore. It should take into account:

- Sensitivity of the clitoris
- Size of the clitoris
- Sensitivity of the labia
- Style of pubic hair
- G-spot sensitivity and penetration preferences

SENSITIVITY OF THE CLITORIS

The clitoris varies greatly in its response to stimulation. Some females prefer intense stimulation while others find anything other than indirect stimulation to be excessive, even painful. As such, it is worth following a scale of stimulation, starting at the lowest level and only progressing at the request—whether verbal or nonverbal—of the female in question. It is far better to understimulate a partner, making her beg for additional stimulation, than to kill the mood with overenthusiastic and pain-inducing techniques (see *She Won't Tell You, But She Will Tell Her Friends: Female Response to Poor Male Sexual Technique*, by Dr. Honor Bound).

EXTREMELY SENSITIVE CLITORIS. Focus attention on the labia and pubic mound, avoiding the clitoris entirely. Indirect stimulation may be applied by licking around the clitoris in large circles. However, care should be taken to avoid accidental contact, factoring in movements of the female. Holding the hips down to ensure that the woman remains static may help minimize this risk. Gaffer's tape is not to be recommended, as it is liable to cause chafing.

A soft approach is by far the most beneficial, and also provides a good starting position for cunnilingus with a new partner. Simply breathing on the labia and clitoris, or dribbling onto the clitoris, may provide enough stimulation for climax.

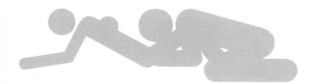

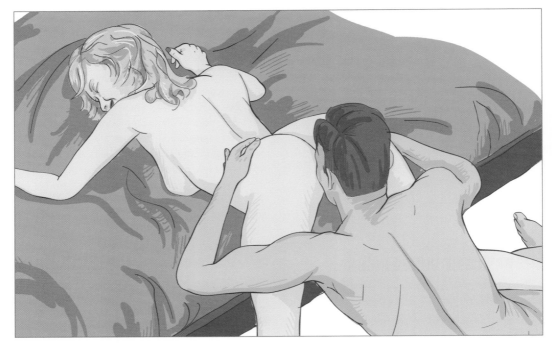

Figure 1: Use the hands to caress the body while performing oral coitus.

Note: A woman with a sensitive clitoris may need additional relaxation prior to oral stimulation due to fears of a pain response. Massage is the ideal form of initial foreplay, helping soothe a mate in a caring and appropriate way. Groping the buttocks while massaging a partner will belie your intent.

SENSITIVE CLITORIS. Use the side or underside of the tongue to stimulate the clitoris, rather than the tip of the tongue. This limits the amount of pressure on the clitoris, while still allowing for creativity.

Cupping the pubic mound with the entire hand and gently rocking will give less direct clitoral stimulation, which may be more palatable for a mate.

Approach the vagina from behind, focus on the outer and inner labia, and use the tongue to penetrate the vagina to provide pleasurable sensation without risk of inadvertent clitoral stimulation.

RESPONSIVE CLITORIS. Using the tip of the tongue in addition to the side of the tongue for stimulation will ensure the student can target sensation in a precise fashion. Lapping, sucking, and licking can all reap rewards, while manual stimulation may add extra sensation.

Toys may also be incorporated into oral-genital coitus, but are not absolutely required. However, the seminal paper *Fast Food Foreplay: How the Vibrator Revolutionized Heterosexual Sex Lives*, by Dr. Buzz Aughton, is highly recommended, particularly if the student fears that a lack of stamina may inhibit performance.

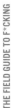

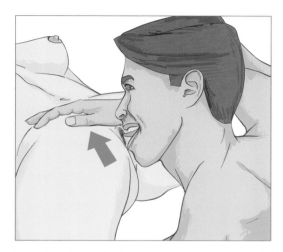

Figure 2: Pushing the heel of the hand into the pubic mound will retract the clitoral hood.

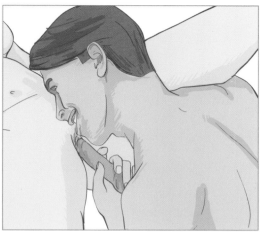

Figure 3: Manual penetration or toy–based penetration can add extra pleasure to cunnilingus.

MILDLY INSENSITIVE CLITORIS. Pressing the heel of the hand into the pubic mound will help retract the clitoral hood, exposing the clitoral tip to allow for more intense stimulation. Suction can increase blood flow to the area, thus boosting sensitivity. Combining manual stimulation with oral stimulation is a must.

Toys are an optional addition to the proceedings.

EXTREMELY INSENSITIVE CLITORIS. Using a vibrator during cunnilingus can help increase levels of stimulation. If a partner is extremely clitorally insensitive, opt for a high-power vibrating bullet rather than a standard vibrator. Team this with clitoral suction and, with permission, gentle nibbling.

In extreme cases, and only with permission, spanking the area prior to commencing cunnilingus will help fire up the nerve endings, again boosting blood flow and increasing sensitivity.

SIZE OF THE CLITORIS
It is impossible to project expectations about a woman's clitoral size based on any factor other than whether she has given birth. Instead, ensure that you allow plenty of time for exploration prior to commencing cunnilingus.

INVISIBLE CLITORIS. Although the comedic profession has taken to mocking males who are unable to locate the clitoris, some women have a clitoral bud that is nearly impossible to find. This is particularly common in obese women, as the additional fat layers in the pubic mound can mask the clitoris, making it appear smaller than it is.

When faced with an invisible clitoris, it is best to seek guidance from the subject. Manual self-stimulation by the subject will indicate the area that should be focused on during oral stimulation. For best results, this self-stimulation should be maintained for the duration of oral-genital congress.

SMALL CLITORIS. A small clitoris should be approached in a similar way to an invisible one. However, it may also be possible to locate the clitoris by manually spreading the labia, to allow a more graphic view of the genitals. Utilizing toys or suction (assuming the small clitoris is not of the sensitive variety) will greatly aid progress, because the clitoris swells during arousal, making it easier to identify.

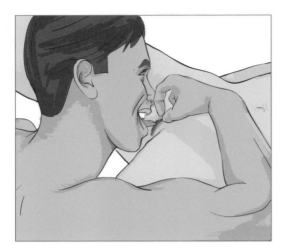

Figure 4: If a woman has a less than sensitive clitoris, gently pinching it can increase blood flow to the area, and subsequent pleasure.

MEDIUM CLITORIS. If the clitoris is of average size, there is no excuse for neglecting it. Trace the tongue up both the left and the right side of the clitoris: most women have a preference for a left- or right-biased approach, though many will never have explored t his and will thus reap great rewards from a partner's superior knowledge. Similarly, flickering the tongue both up and down and from side to side, and monitoring response accordingly, will help identify a woman's oral-genital stimulation preferences.

LARGE CLITORIS. A woman with a large clitoris may feel self-conscious, but it allows for a wider array of cunnilingus techniques. Sucking the entire clitoris into the mouth and flickering the tongue over the clitoral tip can provide intense stimulation, assuming that the large clitoris is not also of the highly sensitive variety. With an extremely large clitoris, using the fingers to masturbate the shaft of the clitoris while the tongue explores the clitoral tip can lead to intense orgasmic satisfaction.

SENSITIVITY OF THE LABIA

As with the clitoris, labial sensitivity can vary greatly from woman to woman. However, as a general rule, the outer labia (labia majora) are less sensitive than the inner labia (labia minora). In addition, the labia minora may become more highly sensitized as a result of increased estrogen levels (for example, due to using the contraceptive pill).

The labia may also vary in size, with racial factors feeding into genital structure. Some women have labia minora that project beyond the labia majora. However, this is no cause for concern and has little bearing on oral-genital congress, unless it leads to feelings of insecurity in the female mate. If so, praising the genital structure can help ease relaxation and capacity for climax.

EXTREMELY SENSITIVE LABIA. If the labia are extremely sensitive, approaching them with the side or underside of the tongue will help ensure that oral-genital congress is pleasurable rather than painful. Breathing over the labia—but not up the vagina, which can be dangerous—may also give sufficient stimulation.

SENSITIVE LABIA. Sensitive labia can be a boon in oral-genital congress, offering a "second clitoris" to stimulate. Teaming gentle manual stimulation with oral pleasuring will reap an optimal response.

RESPONSIVE LABIA. Licking the inner labia, gently sucking the outer labia into the mouth, and sucking the clitoris present a well-rounded approach to cunnilingus. Using the fingers to softly squeeze the labia while the tongue focuses on the clitoris may increase pleasure for the female study partner.

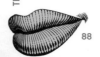

TRACE THE TONGUE UP BOTH THE LEFT AND THE RIGHT SIDE OF THE CLITORIS: MOST WOMEN HAVE A PREFERENCE FOR A LEFT- OR RIGHT-BIASED APPROACH, THOUGH MANY WILL NEVER HAVE EXPLORED THIS AND WILL THUS REAP GREAT REWARDS FROM A PARTNER'S SUPERIOR KNOWLEDGE.

MILDLY INSENSITIVE LABIA. As with an insensitive clitoris, insensitive labia can be effectively stimulated with toys. Opt for a butterfly-style vibrating device that attaches to the body with a harness and provides vibration to the labia and clitoris. Adding a tongue to the equation is likely to thrill an experimental partner.

EXTREMELY INSENSITIVE LABIA. Shaving the pubic area can heighten sensitivity. As such, it may help increase stimulation to the area, particularly if teamed with labial squeezing, pinching, or slapping (with consent). As with an extremely insensitive clitoris, extremely insensitive labia may respond well to a high-revolution vibrating bullet.

STYLE OF PUBIC HAIR

Pubic hair has become a fashion accessory for women, with ethnographic studies indicating pubic hair styles as diverse as the "Tiffany," a small square of pubic hair dyed duck-egg blue, and the "Landing Strip," a rectangle of short hair that indicates the approach route to the vagina. Although these minor variations have little impact on oral-genital congress, the broad subcategories may have an influence on labial sensitivity.

FULLY SHAVEN. Also referred to as a Brazilian or the Hollywood, a fully shaven pubic area is ideal for oral-genital congress, offering full scope for exploration. Lapping the pubic mound and upper labia majora, in addition to the clitoris and labia minora, offers a unique form of stimulation that takes maximum advantage of the defoliated state of a female study partner.

SHAPED. Most pubic hair shaping entails removing all but the hair visible on the pubic mound, which is then trimmed into shapes such as a heart, lightning bolt, or square. This leaves the lower labia free of hair and in an optimal state to be sucked.

TRIMMED. Simply trimming the hair to keep it tidy is still a popular option with many women, being both well groomed and low maintenance. Brushing through the pubic hair will help ensure errant hairs do not limit activity. The pubic hair can also be kept soft with the occasional application of conditioner. When approaching a natural woman, it may be necessary to part the labia majora manually to ensure that hair is kept out of the way and to ease visibility.

NATURAL. Allowing the pubic hair to maintain its natural shape is often stigmatized in current culture, because of media (in particular, adult media) depictions of female beauty. However, a natural pubic area is nothing to be ashamed of, as long as it is clean and regularly brushed. It may present a challenge for the earnest sexual explorer who has to fight through the hair. However, parting the labia majora will ease the path, allowing the tongue free access. Gently tugging on the pubic hair can also be pleasurable.

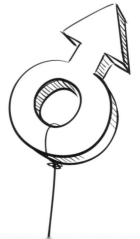

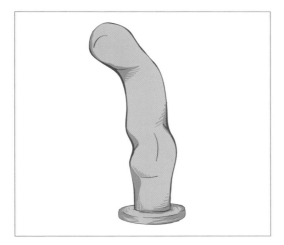

Figure 5: A curved toy will help you reach the G-spot.

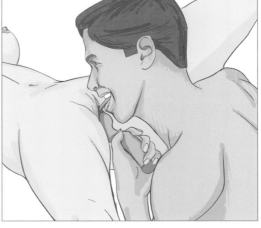

Figure 6: Teaming a toy with G-spot stimulation offers an intense experience.

G-SPOT SENSITIVITY

Although penetration is core to the heterosexual act of coitus, it is of greater pleasure to a man than a woman, as the majority of nerve endings in the vagina are focused at the entrance. However, some women have a sensitive G-spot (see chapter 1) that can provide an additional method of stimulation during oral-genital congress.

LITTLE OR NO G-SPOT RESPONSE. Some women report little G-spot response, or are unable to locate the G-spot at all. As such, penetration is less likely to be of key consideration, and oral-genital contact should focus on clitoral and labial exploration.

MILD G-SPOT RESPONSE. If a female study partner enjoys G-spot stimulation, combining internal manual stimulation with external clitoral stimulation will demonstrate a keen understanding of oral-genital technique. Bend the top knuckle of the finger and use this to press into the G-spot, which should swell in response.

The uninitiated scholar may be surprised by a flood of liquid, should the woman concerned be trained in female ejaculation techniques, which is something that should be taken into consideration to avoid any surprises. Female ejaculate is perfectly safe to ingest but may be copious in some women.

EXTREME G-SPOT RESPONSE. Should G-spot stimulation be of key importance to a female mate, it may be worth considering using technology to assist your endeavors, as maintaining G-spot stimulation manually for an extended period of time may be tiring.

There are numerous toys designed with G-spot stimulation in mind, most of which have a crooked tip. These should be positioned by the female subject initially, because, unlike with manual stimulation, it can be difficult to locate the G-spot with a toy. Teaming stimulation of the G-spot using a toy with clitoral stimulation using the tongue is an act that will mark a scholar as being extremely advanced.

TEAMING STIMULATION OF THE G-SPOT USING A TOY WITH CLITORAL STIMULATION USING THE TONGUE IS AN ACT THAT WILL MARK A SCHOLAR AS BEING EXTREMELY ADVANCED.

THE BASICS OF FELLATIO

The optimal fellatio technique should take into account the following:

- Size of the penis
- Sensitivity of the penis
- Presence or absence of foreskin
- Sensitivity of the testicles

In addition, psychosexual desires should be considered when determining whether to assume a dominant, neutral, or submissive stance.

SIZE OF THE PENIS

Many men feel insecure about the size of their penis and wish to be better endowed. The following information should be used for educational purposes and should not instill any feelings of ego deflation.

SMALL PENIS. For the purposes of fellatio, a small penis offers infinitely more options. It can be sucked into the mouth in full, and deep throat should be eminently possible assuming that the female scholar has suitably prepared her gag reflex. Indeed, with a small enough penis, the gag reflex may not even come into play.

Using fingers rather than an entire hand to masturbate the shaft during oral sex will help ensure that the male subject feels more well endowed than he is, which can provide a valuable psychological edge and speed climax.

MEDIUM PENIS. A medium-size member also offers itself up to multiple forms of oral stimulation. It can be sucked into the mouth or throat, licked all over, and stimulated with a flickering tongue over the head while the hand focuses on the shaft and testicles.

LARGE PENIS. Handling a large penis during oral sex can be challenging. Gag reflex training is essential, and the female scholar may find it easiest to initiate oral congress from a flaccid state to allow the mouth to get used to the sensation. If the penis is too large to take comfortably into the mouth, licking the glans while stroking the shaft can offer an alternative to fellatio, as can encouraging the male research partner to masturbate into the female's mouth while she flickers her tongue over the head of the penis. If deep throating is impossible, it can be simulated by aiming the head of the penis into the side of the cheek.

SENSITIVITY OF THE PENIS

As with the female sexual structure, the male genital region can vary massively in sensitivity. This can lead to premature or retarded ejaculation, and will also have an effect on the amount of time it takes from initiating oral congress to stimulating a research partner to climax.

Enhancing Coital Technique by Removing Genital-Centricity

In addition to the criteria in this chapter, students of sexual techniques should consider peripheral enhancements to cunnilingus. These include:

THIGH STIMULATION. The inner thighs can be highly sensitive. Licking, biting, and gently scratching the area as a prequel to oral sex can help build anticipation while also providing a useful key to a partner's levels of response. This also allows the keen student extra study time to analyze the genital region prior to commencing oral-genital contact.

BREAST STIMULATION. Caressing the nipples and breasts while administering cunnilingus can add an extra level of pleasure. This can be particularly effective with a partner who has an extremely sensitive clitoris, as nipple stimulation can send pleasurable signals to the clitoris without directly stimulating the nerve endings.

MENTAL STIMULATION. Interspersing oral contact with erotic whispers can help intensify sensation. As such, it is a particularly valuable addition to proceedings with a partner who lacks sensitivity in the clitoris, labia, or both. However, this lack of sensitivity should not be assumed to extend to the mind: a woman with a sensitive clitoris is no more likely to find appeal in the phrase, "Suck my love stick, you cheap trollop," than one with a more responsive nubbin.

ADDITIONAL AIDS. Champagne, mouthwash, and tingling lubricants can all add extra sensation to cunnilingus. As such, they are valuable tools to use on a partner with lesser sensitivity in the genital region. However, should sugar be used in the area (such as the sugars in alcohol) it is essential to wash thoroughly after climax to minimize the risk of *Candida albicans* (commonly referred to as a yeast infection or thrush).

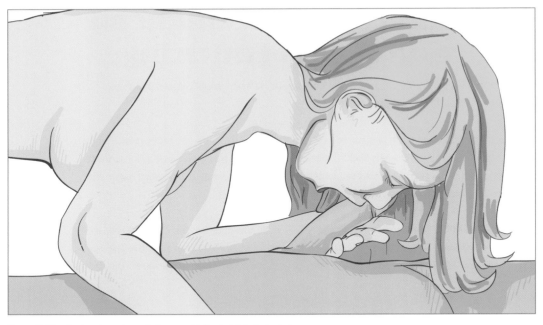

Figure 7: Use the hands and mouth for a sophisticated fellatio technique.

EXTREMELY SENSITIVE PENIS. Stimulating an extremely sensitive penis may be painful if it is too enthusiastic. To minimize the risk, focus attention on the shaft of the penis rather than the glans, and avoid touching or licking the frenulum unless specifically asked to do so. Keep suction light and even, and use the flat of the tongue, rather than the tip, to lap at the penis. Minimize use of the hand unless you want to speed climax and, if applied, keep it purely on the shaft rather than the glans.

SENSITIVE PENIS. A sensitive penis is liable to ejaculate rapidly. Therefore, minimize foreplay prior to administering oral sex to ensure that there is enough time for the male to enjoy the act of oral coitus. Varying techniques will encourage a sensitive partner to last longer. Speeding climax is easy: apply regular rhythmic, gentle sucking and, if that fails to generate climax, add a hand to the equation.

RESPONSIVE PENIS. A responsive penis can be handled with a little less reticence, though equal care and attention are obviously required. Combine oral stimulation with manual stimulation, and let the tongue swirl around the glans, then flicker over the head with every thrust. Alternate soft sucking with more vigorous head bobbing for optimal results.

MILDLY INSENSITIVE PENIS. Some men require a little more stimulation to reach climax. Alcohol, drugs, and certain medical conditions can affect this as well.

If a man lacks penile sensitivity, it is worth spending time on additional foreplay prior to commencing fellatio, or it may lead to an aching mouth. Rapid head bobbing and deep-throating techniques will give extra stimulation and increase the likelihood of ejaculation occurring before the onset of lockjaw.

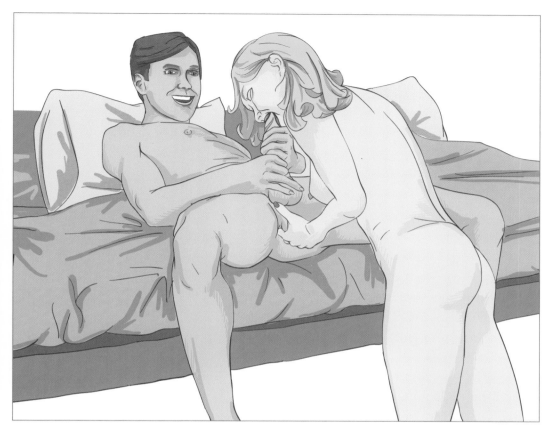

Figure 8: Simultaneous masturbation offers an easy way to speed climax through oral sex.

EXTREMELY INSENSITIVE PENIS. An extremely insensitive penis can require significant stimulation before climax is reached, if it can be reached at all. Therefore, initiate plenty of foreplay prior to administering fellatio. Paying attention to visual elements may also be of use, as men are often visually led. Looking a mate in the eye while fellating him or caressing one's own breasts may provide an additional frisson and help speed climax. Asking a partner to masturbate while oral sex is being administered can also be effective. Prostate stimulation can intensify sensation, should the research partner be suitably experimental.

PRESENCE OR ABSENCE OF FORESKIN

Although some researchers claim that an uncircumcised penis is unclean, in reality, the presence or absence of foreskin is simply a cultural practice. Removing the foreskin doesn't enhance sex and may even lead to loss of sensation. As such, it is important to consider a research partner's foreskin status prior to commencing oral-genital congress.

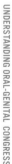

CIRCUMCISED PENIS. A circumcised penis is likely to be less sensitive than an uncircumcised one, because the glans of the penis is constantly exposed to friction through rubbing against a man's clothes. As such, it should be treated accordingly.

The circumcised penis is also likely to self-lubricate to a lesser degree. It is worth using lubricant, whether artificial or natural, before commencing manual stimulation, or chafing may result. It is well worth keeping a glass of water at hand to ensure that saliva levels can be maintained throughout.

UNCIRCUMCISED PENIS. An uncircumcised penis may smell a little more strongly than a circumcised one, because the foreskin must be pushed back to wash underneath it. As such, the novice researcher may wish to initiate a shared bath or shower prior to instigating oral congress. If the issue is comparatively minor, it can be dealt with using a generous amount of saliva to dilute the taste instead. Pushing the foreskin back and forth over the glans can provide exquisite stimulation, particularly when teamed with a tongue flickering underneath the foreskin.

SENSITIVITY OF THE TESTICLES

The testicles are often neglected in oral-genital congress. However, some men find testicle stimulation an intensely pleasurable addition to fellatio.

SENSITIVE TESTICLES. If a man's testicles are sensitive, it may be worth ignoring them altogether. However, with a gentle enough approach, licking or stroking the testicles as part of oral-genital congress may provide extra frisson. Go slowly and avoid sucking the testicles unless actively requested to do so, as this may be too intense for the recipient.

RESPONSIVE TESTICLES. Responsive testicles can be stroked, cupped, gently tugged, and sucked into the mouth (in an act colloquially referred to as "teabagging" because of the dipping motion used by a male straddling a female's face).

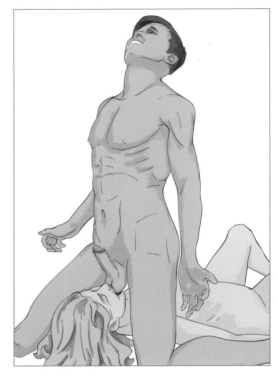

Figure 9: Teabagging: so called because the testicles are dipped into the woman's mouth.

Some men enjoy feeling both testicles being sucked into the mouth at once while others prefer solo testicle suction. Keep all suction gentle and handle with care, because the testicles are highly sensitive even if they are responsive, and bruising the testicles is all too easy. Licking the testicles can provide a visual thrill for the male research subject, in addition to a pleasurable sensation.

INSENSITIVE TESTICLES. With insensitive testicles, it may be worth focusing attention on the penis. However, light tugging, suction, and gentle squeezing may be pleasurable. Don't squeeze hard, though, because no matter how insensitive the testicles may be, it is all too easy to damage them.

Adding Sophistication to Male Seduction

In addition to the criteria in this chapter, students of sexual techniques should consider peripheral enhancements to fellatio. These include:

THIGH STIMULATION. As with women, a man's inner thighs can be highly sensitive. Licking, biting, and gently scratching the area as a prequel to oral sex can provide a sensual tease, allowing anticipation to build before oral-genital congress commences.

NIPPLE STIMULATION. Caressing the nipples isn't something that should be limited to a female partner. Many men have sensitive nipples, too, and gently stroking, squeezing, or pinching them during oral sex may provide pleasurable sensations.

ADDITIONAL AIDS. As with cunnilingus, certain aids can enhance the sensation of fellatio. Ice cubes can be used to cool the mouth—though ice should always be sucked before being used anywhere else on the body, or ice burns may result. Conversely, tea or coffee can be used to warm the mouth, but again, boiling liquids should be avoided. Sparkling drinks such as soda water or Champagne may add sensation and can be particularly useful if a man has an insensitive penis. Adding a cock ring to the base of the penis will trap blood in the penis, thus increasing sensitivity. Should a man enjoy prostate stimulation, the use of a butt plug may speed climax.

ENCOUNTERING ANOMALIES IN ORAL-GENITAL CONGRESS

Should you encounter piercings during oral-genital congress, consider the following oral sex techniques and contraindications (return to chapter 1 should you require clarification as to the nature of any piercings). Obviously, no new piercings should be orally stimulated until they have fully healed.

MALE PIERCINGS

PRINCE ALBERT/REVERSE PRINCE ALBERT. This can be softly sucked to increase sensation during oral-genital congress. However, extreme suction must not be applied because of the risk of tearing.

SHAFT AMPALLANG. Take care to avoid accidentally knocking this piercing, should manual manipulation be employed during fellatio. Softly sucking the piercing may be pleasurable.

TRANSCROTAL PIERCING. Don't employ heavy suction to the testicles during oral-genital congress.

DYDOE. This can be gently flicked with the tongue to add extra sensation during fellatio.

FRENULUM PIERCING. Soft licking will be intensely pleasurable, but hard suction should be avoided to decrease risk of tearing.

GUICHE PIERCING. This tends to respond well to licking and sucking. Softly pressing it with a tongue or finger while administering oral pleasure may also prove effective.

FEMALE PIERCINGS

CLITORAL HOOD PIERCING. Soft sucking will indirectly stimulate the clitoris, but harder suction should be avoided to minimize the risk of tearing.

CLITORIS PIERCING. Care should be taken, and hard suction only employed upon request.

CHRISTINA PIERCING. Focusing on the clitoris is likely to ensure one's study partner removes the piercing in a timely fashion, allowing access to the vagina.

LABIAL PIERCING. Again, plenty of clitoral stimulation should speed its removal.

FOURCHETTE PIERCING. Licking the piercing or softly pressing it in with one's tongue can enhance pleasure during oral-genital congress.

TRIANGLE PIERCING. This is the only genital piercing that can stimulate the clitoris from behind, making it ideal for enhancing rear-entry cunnilingus.

ANALYZING AND HONING THE EFFECTIVENESS OF YOUR APPROACH

With correct study of your research partner's genitals and appropriate stimulation based on the characteristics that you have identified, climax through oral-genital congress should be relatively easy to achieve. To advance to the next chapter, please ensure you have:

- Stimulated a research partner orally to climax
- Used primary and secondary erogenous zones to enhance the sensation for the research partner
- Explored the use of oral-genital congress aids
- Familiarized yourself with anomalies that may be encountered in the field (extra credit for research conducted in the field)

Once this level of comprehension has been achieved, you may progress to coitus.

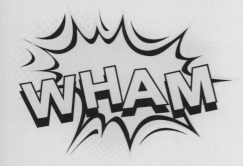

Chapter 5:

Coitus Complexitus Improvedicus

AVAILABLE OPTIONS IN PENETRATIVE VAGINAL COITUS

After sufficient study of the precoital arts, the dedicated student may progress to coitus complexitus, often deemed the loftiest of sexual acts. Indeed, some people claim that it is only coitus complexitus that qualifies as "sex," with all other contact being merely a precursor to the act.

This is a sexually unsophisticated view, but it is certainly true to say that copulation can offer some of the finest sexual pleasures known to humankind. The sensation of the phallus entering the vagina is compelling—as it should be, given that the survival of the human race depends upon it. However, it is here more than in any other sex act that genital compatibility comes into play.

While an act of coupling between two people who share a mutual attraction is liable to be pleasurable, there are numerous issues that can be avoided by ensuring that the genitals are suitably matched. Should you find a partner with complementary genitals to your own, all positions outlined in this chapter are within your scope. If not, using the appropriate positions and props will help ensure a more satisfactory outcome.

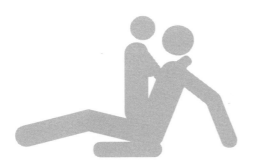

MINIMIZING RISK FACTORS IN LESS COMPATIBLE GENITAL PAIRINGS

The course of true love does not always run smooth, as Shakespeare noted. However, should an affection develop between two people with less compatible genitals, the following guidelines may help achieve a mutually pleasurable outcome.

SMALL VAGINA/LARGE PENIS

Penetration of the vagina can be extremely uncomfortable if the male is of larger dimensions than the female can easily accept. However, effective foreplay can help minimize this issue. Ensure that at least twenty minutes of foreplay are administered prior to attempting penetration, and only do so at the behest of the female.

Lubrication is essential to ease entry. A significant level of precoital exploration may be enough to generate this naturally in the woman. However, bottled lubricant may be required, particularly if the male is extremely well endowed.

The optimal position for this genital combination is woman on top, as this allows the female to set the pace. Under no circumstance should the male attempt to push the woman deeper onto the phallus by placing his hands on her hips. Instead, he should allow the female to ease her way onto him, letting her vagina relax to assist entry.

IT IS HERE MORE THAN IN ANY OTHER SEX ACT THAT GENITAL COMPATIBILITY COMES INTO PLAY.

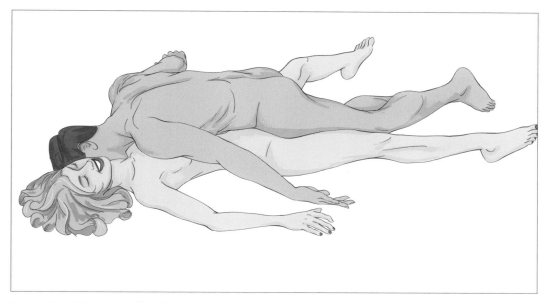

Figure 1: The CAT technique offers clitoral stimulation and can greatly increase a woman's chance of orgasm.

Should the woman lean backward, this will deepen penetration; care is advised. Conversely, leaning forward will offer clitoral stimulation and is recommended.

Missionary position can also work well for this pairing. However, the woman should keep her legs flat on the bed rather than raising them, to ensure that penetration levels are limited. Coital alignment technique (also known as CAT), in which the man lies flat on top of the woman, with his hips parallel to hers, his phallus inside her, and the base of his penis rubbing against the clitoris, is reported to increase a woman's chance of climax by around 70 percent. If attempting the CAT position, the male should rock back and forth rather than thrusting in the usual fashion, as this increases clitoral stimulation.

LARGE VAGINA/SMALL PENIS
A man with a small penis may find that friction is lacking during coitus with a woman who has a large vagina. This may be alleviated if the woman practices Kegel exercises on a regular basis and flexes her vaginal muscles during sex. In addition, positions that allow the woman to put her legs together will help tighten the vagina.

Flat doggy-style sex, in which the woman lies on her front, facedown, and allows the man to penetrate her from the rear, is a good position for this pairing. The positive effects can be enhanced if the woman crosses her legs once the male has entered her.

Similarly, standard doggy, with the woman on all fours, can also allow the woman to cross her legs after penetration, with the advantage that this position optimizes depth of penetration.

COITUS COMPLEXITUS IMPROVEDICUS

Should the female require more stimulation, using a butt plug or vibrator inside the vagina alongside the penis will help tighten the vagina, thus enhancing the experience for both parties. However, this should only be attempted should both parties be curious about the sensation, as it may be a little extreme for some people.

SMALL CLITORIS/SMALL PENIS

While a large penis will stretch the vagina, thus pulling the clitoral hood down over the clitoris to provide indirect stimulation, a small penis is unlikely to do so. As such, clitoral stimulation must be attempted in some other way.

CAT is likely to be pleasurable for both parties (see Small Vagina/Large Penis for details). Alternatively, rear-entry sex allows either party easy access to the clitoris either manually or with a vibrator.

SENSITIVE CLITORIS/INSENSITIVE PENIS

A sensitive clitoris may find the extended coitus required by an insensitive penis to be painful. Therefore, it is worth spending a significant amount of time on precoital pleasuring to ensure that the male is as close to climax as possible.

Rear-entry positions allow stimulation of the penis without providing clitoral stimulation. Should the female dislike deep penetration, flat doggy style, in which the woman lies on her front rather than kneeling on all fours, offers a suitable alternative to standard doggy style.

Standing sex may also appeal; here, the woman stands facing the wall with her arms braced against it, and the man penetrates from behind. Penetration can be deepened if the woman bends her torso farther forward. Crossing the legs in either of these positions will increase stimulation for the male. However, it will also give indirect stimulation to the clitoris, so it should be avoided if the woman is extremely sensitive.

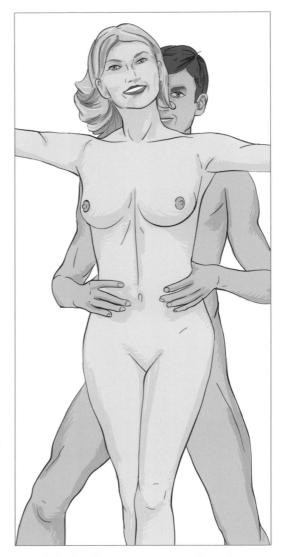

Figure 2: Sex from the rear deepens penetration and may assist with an insensitive penis.

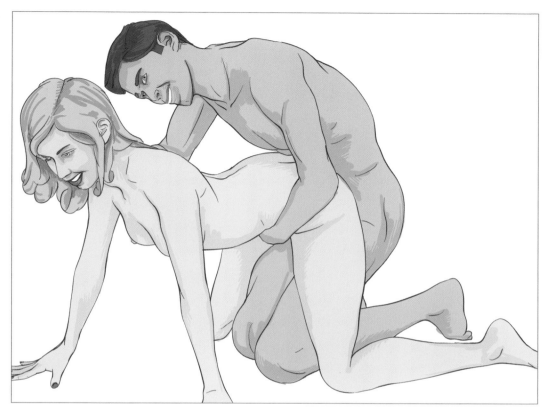

Figure 3: Doggy-style sex offers animal passion and allows easy access for either manual or toy-based stimulation.

To increase stimulation of the penis, the woman should flex her Kegel muscles. The male may find it beneficial to wear a cock ring to trap blood in the penis and ensure a maximum erection level is achieved.

INSENSITIVE CLITORIS/SENSITIVE PENIS

Conversely, if the female has an insensitive clitoris, she will require significant foreplay to ensure that she reaches climax with a male who has a sensitive penis. His precoital pleasuring should be kept to a minimum to ensure that he is erect but not significantly aroused.

CAT allows maximum clitoral stimulation (see Small Vagina/Large Penis for details). Alternatively, doggy-style sex with the woman's legs spread wide will limit friction to the penis while allowing easy access for manual or toy-based clitoral stimulation.

LARGE PENIS/FEMALE WHO DISLIKES DEEP PENETRATION

A male with a large penis needs to take care not to hurt his partner. Vaginal bruising is easily done with hard thrusting and can lead to cystitis and other disorders. To minimize this risk, woman-on-top positions are recommended.

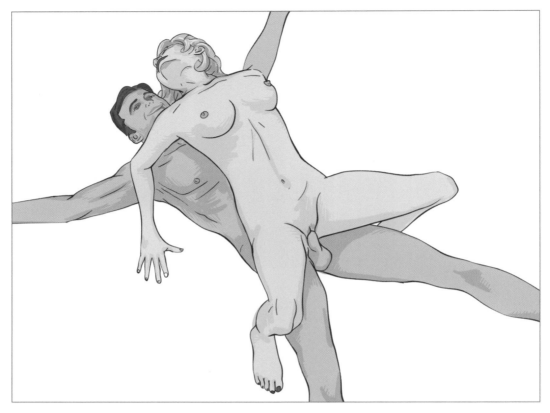

Figure 4: Reverse cowgirl will make the smallest man feel bigger—as long as he doesn't slip out.

Rear-entry positions allow for deep penetration and should be avoided unless the woman is in control. This is most easily possible in the starfish position, in which the male lies with his legs spread and the woman lies on top of him, face up, having first squatted over the male to allow his penis to enter her vagina, then leaned back until she is lying on top of his body.

Sideways sex can also be ideal, if both parties face each other, as this minimizes the length of the penis that can easily penetrate the vagina.

SMALL PENIS/FEMALE WHO LIKES DEEP PENETRATION

If a female requires deeper penetration than the male's phallus can provide, rear-entry sex is advised, with standard doggy style being the most effective variation. Penetration can be further deepened when a woman is on all fours if she arches her back or uses her hands against the headboard to push herself back onto her partner.

In missionary position, putting a cushion under the buttocks will help deepen penetration, and to further increase the depth, raising the legs will also help. The higher the legs are raised, the deeper penetration will be.

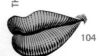

THE MAJORITY OF COUPLES HAVE SEX IN ONLY THREE DIFFERENT SEXUAL POSITIONS, WITH LITTLE VARIATION, ONCE THEY HAVE ESTABLISHED A MUTUALLY BENEFICIAL FORM OF CONGRESS. SIMPLY ADAPTING THESE POSITIONS IN MINOR WAYS CAN HELP REFRESH A TIRED RELATIONSHIP AND REIGNITE EARLY FLAMES OF PASSION.

TAINTED LOVE: COPING WITH NONGENITAL INCOMPATIBILITIES

Coitus is not merely a matter of engaging genitals. There are also numerous other incompatibilities that should be taken into account for optimal intercourse.

HEAVY MALE/LIGHT FEMALE

Although it is common for a male to be heavier than a female, if the size differential is significant, this can make positions such as missionary uncomfortable for the female. Further, obesity can make the penis seem smaller due to fat in the pubic mound shortening the usable length of the penis. Thus, rear-entry sex is best, either in the form of doggy style or standing sex, as this allows maximum penetration while also ensuring the male can support his own weight. Woman on top is also worth considering if the male is sufficiently well endowed.

HEAVY FEMALE/LIGHT MALE

If a woman is significantly larger than her partner, this may make entry inconvenient in the missionary position. However, the woman can lie on the bed with her legs spread at the edge, and the male can stand or kneel between her legs to penetrate her. Rear entry offers another option, though the woman may need to part her buttocks to allow maximum penetration.

ORGASMIC MALE/LESS ORGASMIC FEMALE

It is far from uncommon that the male finds it easier to climax than the female does. However, it is optimal to ensure that both partners reach orgasm during sex, or resentment can build up. Extended foreplay for the female is a must. The CAT position provides maximum stimulation to the clitoris, and it is well worth incorporating manual or toy-based stimulation into coitus. A butterfly-style vibrator that fastens around the thighs will provide clitoral stimulation while leaving both partners' hands free to stimulate the woman's primary and secondary erogenous zones.

LESS ORGASMIC MALE/ORGASMIC FEMALE

Although women generally take longer to achieve climax than men do, there are some women for whom orgasm is easy. This can be a limiting factor during sex if her partner finds it harder to reach climax, as the vagina tends to get both wetter and looser after climax, thus reducing friction. To counter this, the female should extend precoital contact until the male is nearing climax. In addition, rear-entry positions that allow deep penetration but limited clitoral stimulation will provide a dual-pronged approach. Regular Kegel exercises will help the woman maintain vaginal tightness post-climax.

REMOVING A SENSE OF ENNUI FROM TRADITIONAL COITAL POSITIONS

Even with a correct genital pairing, after repeated acts of coitus, it is possible that disillusionment with the act may occur. This is due partly to the gradual diminishing of the chemicals that first attract potential mates to each other and partly to a lack of experimentation that often signifies later stages in a couple's relationship. The majority of couples have sex in only three different sexual positions, with little variation, once they have established a mutually beneficial form of congress. Simply adapting these positions in minor ways can help refresh a tired relationship and reignite early flames of passion.

MISSIONARY POSITION VARIATIONS

Missionary position, in which the male lies on top of the female, is generally believed to be the most commonly used sexual position. This is unsurprising by dint of the fact that it allows stimulation of the clitoris and penetration of varying depths.

To deepen penetration, place pillows underneath the hips. If the woman raises one or both legs in the air, this will also increase the depth to which her partner may thrust. It is worth experimenting with raising the right and the left leg individually because changing the angle of entry will also change the way that coitus feels for both partners.

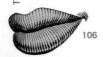

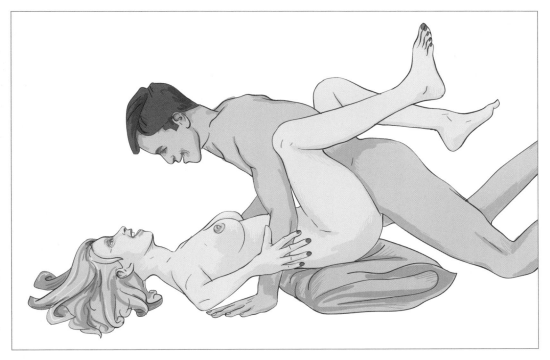

Figure 5: Raising the legs will help angle the penis toward the G-spot.

The male can vary missionary position by raising himself up to different levels. Lying flat on top of the woman allows maximum intimacy but may limit the woman's breathing if maintained for a significant amount of time. Raising himself up on his forearms allows greater traction and increased penetration.

To gain maximum penetration, the woman can lie with her legs hanging over the edge of the bed and the male can kneel or stand between her thighs, raising her legs to rest on his shoulders.

Looking a lover in the eyes during missionary sex may seem like a minimal change, but if you have never tried it before, you may be surprised by the intensity that it can add to coitus.

REAR-ENTRY VARIATIONS

Traditionally viewed as a more "animal" sexual position than missionary position, rear entry offers myriad variations. Some women may feel concerned about the lack of intimacy (and indeed, some males dislike being unable to look their partner in the eyes during coitus). To counter this issue, try rear-entry coitus while standing in front of a mirror. This allows you to look at each other and gives a voyeuristic thrill to the male, who can watch his hands exploring his lover's body or enjoy the sight of the woman's breasts.

Rear-entry sex offers the deepest penetration. However, there is immense variation of sensation based on the angle of entry. If both parties lie flat, penetration is lessened but clitoral stimulation can be easily provided through manual stimulation or by the

TRY REAR-ENTRY COITUS WHILE STANDING IN FRONT OF A MIRROR. THIS ALLOWS YOU TO LOOK AT EACH OTHER AND GIVES A VOYEURISTIC THRILL TO THE MALE, WHO CAN WATCH HIS HANDS EXPLORING HIS LOVER'S BODY OR ENJOY THE SIGHT OF THE WOMAN'S BREASTS.

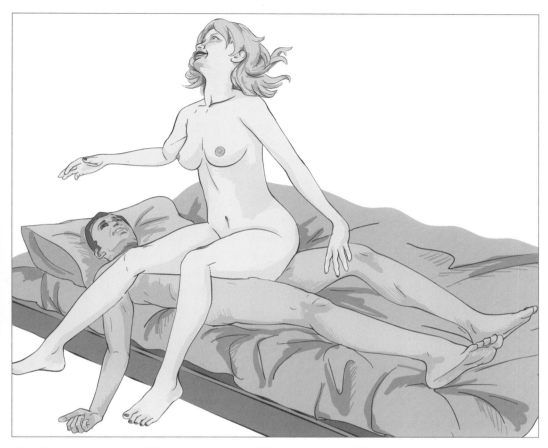

Figure 6: For a more unusual position, the female can sit astride her partner sidesaddle.

woman rubbing herself against the mattress. If the woman positions herself on all fours, penetration will be deeper, and this is enhanced if she arches her back.

For increased G-spot stimulation, the woman can kneel instead, with the male kneeling behind her. The woman's balance may be assisted, and extra stimulation gained, if the man supports her by cupping her breasts with his hands.

Rear-entry sex is also ideal for sex in the shower, and allows the woman to spray her clitoris with the shower nozzle for additional stimulation. However,

extra lubrication may be required because water washes away natural juices, particularly when combined with soap.

WOMAN-ON-TOP VARIATIONS
Coitus with the female in the dominant position stimulates different areas depending on the direction in which the woman faces. If she straddles the male with her head toward his feet, in a position known as reverse cowgirl, woman on top offers deep penetration and G-spot stimulation. However, overenthusiastic bucking may lead to discomfort in the male.

COITUS COMPLEXITUS IMPROVEDICUS

If the woman faces the man's head, she can easily lean forward to stimulate her clitoris against the male's pubic mound. It also allows for easy kissing and mutual caressing.

For a more unusual variation of woman-on-top sex, the female can sit astride her partner side-saddle. This position does limit movement, and care must be taken to ensure the penis is not bent at an uncomfortable angle. However, the change in sensation is marked, which may be of particular appeal in a long-term relationship in which all other options have been attempted.

EXTRA CREDIT FOR INCREASED OSTEOPATHIC RISK

In addition, to varying "standard" positions, the keen scholar should experiment with more unusual positions in an effort to ensure that coitus remains exciting. This does not mean that standard coital positions are unable to provide long-term satisfaction or that advanced sexual positions alone will keep coitus optimally satisfying on a long-term basis.

However, only if you fully explore the scope of sexual positions available will you be sure to have tested the delightful array of pleasures of the flesh.

WHEELBARROW

Although this position requires a degree of fitness in both partners, its unusual nature, combined with depth of penetration, means that it offers a memorable experience. The woman should, if possible, do a handstand. (If not, she can lie on the floor). The male should then hold her legs and slowly lower them until her genitals are in line with his. At this point, he should penetrate her, holding on to her legs as he does so. The woman is likely to experience a head rush. Should this become too intense and she starts to feel light-headed, coitus should be stopped to ensure that she does not faint. However, anecdotal evidence suggests that this head rush can enhance the experience for some women.

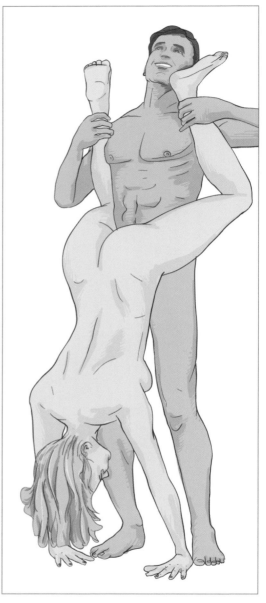

Figure 7: Expect a head rush when trying a standing "69" positon.

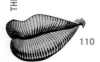

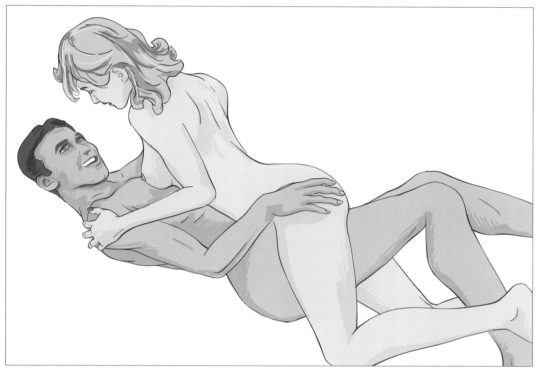

Figure 8: Positions that allow for lots of eye contact build intimacy.

SCISSORS

This position offers optimal clitoral stimulation and deep penetration, though the latter can be limited if the male has a penis that is too large for the female to easily take. Both parties should start in missionary position. Once the male has fully penetrated the female, he should then clasp her around the waist and both parties should move to lie on their sides. The female should then insinuate her lower thigh between the male's legs and place her upper thigh on the male's upper thigh. Her clitoris will now be in direct contact with his thigh, allowing ample flesh for her to grind against. The male can thrust as she does so, giving both parties equal levels of stimulation.

ASSISTED REAR ENTRY

Utilizing furniture is another easy way to enhance or amend coitus. For assisted rear entry, the woman should kneel on a sofa, with her arms and head resting on the back of the sofa. The male can then enter her from behind, kneeling with her torso in between his thighs and his hands resting on the back of the sofa. Both parties can use their hands to increase traction and thus deepen penetration.

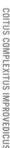

Creation of Sexual Positions for Mutual Benefit

After a thorough comprehension of the subtleties of coitus has been gained, the final stage in understanding coitus complexitus is creating a sexual position that is optimally beneficial to both partners. This not only entails ensuring that genital compatibility is taken into account but also requires using all other skills that have been developed to this point.

Copulation is not an act that benefits from being treated as a sole objective. For truly noteworthy coitus, the keen student should also ensure that secondary erogenous zones are stimulated, whether orally, manually, or with toys. In addition to vibrators, dildos, and clamps, which have been detailed in previous chapters, it is possible to purchase nipple vibrators, scrotal stimulators, and gags (see chapter 8, Advanced Studies for the Impassioned Student, for more information), all of which can be used to take coitus to previously unexplored levels.

In addition, it is worth ensuring that the mind is fully engaged. When considering the position that will deliver the utmost rewards, ensure that you take into account mental as well as physical factors. Does your partner prefer being the dominant or submissive partner? Is stimulation of the nipples effective, or are inner thigh caresses more liable to induce a positive response? You may also wish to consider using aural or visual stimuli to heighten the experience of coitus, whether in the form of talking dirty, watching an adult video, or reading each other highlights from erotic texts.

Do not assume that once coitus commences it should continue as it started. Your partner's physical or psychological preferences may change as coitus progresses. Some women find deep penetration uncomfortable initially but crave more stimulation as they edge nearer to climax. Other people enjoy submissive behavior during the initial stages of coitus but prefer it to become more affectionate and mutual as orgasm approaches.

It is also worth considering the practical. Should either party suffer from back pain, certain positions may be prohibited. Similarly, an unfit student may find certain positions induce fatigue. This is no excuse for sexual laziness, but it is possible to be erotically dexterous without exerting excessive energy. Trailing a sensual hand over a lover's back is unlikely to raise one's cardio-vascular levels, and as such, there is no excuse for its omission, other than a partner's preference.

Conversely, a highly active person may feel unstimulated without multiple position changes in a single act of coitus. Changing positions is one of the key ways to discover new erogenous zones and how to stimulate them, particularly if the parties remain genitally engaged while changing position. However, this should only be attempted with care to ensure the penis is not bent back and the angle of entry does not become uncomfortable for the female.

It is only by repeated experiments that the sexual ideal can be found. This is one of the advantages offered by having a long-term research partner. In addition to providing ample opportunity for practice sessions, a long-term relationship allows couples to develop solid communication techniques. Although a new couple may fear clear discussion of sexual insecurities and issues, a long-established couple is generally all too willing to communicate dissatisfaction with proceedings. Some are so comfortable with their sex lives as to make this amusing dinner party conversation. However, not all guests are comfortable with this level of openness.

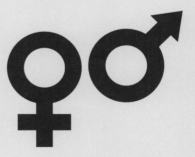

COGNITION AND COITAL PREFERENCES

In addition to size and sensitivity of the genitals, sexual personality plays a part in coitus. For example, a woman with a small vagina may have extremely satisfying sex with a well-endowed man if she is submissive and enjoys extreme levels of stimulation, such as spanking or clamping.

Conversely, a man with a small penis may find sex enjoyable with a woman who has a large vagina if he has a submissive streak and enjoys being sexually humiliated, or has a dominant side and a submissive partner who enjoys dual penetration of the anus and vagina, because this will help tighten the vagina and provide more friction during coitus.

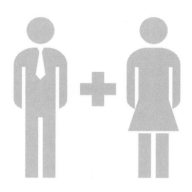

ANALYZING AND HONING THE EFFECTIVENESS OF YOUR APPROACH

Now that coitus has been achieved, the unsophisticated student may assume that the field guide is complete. However, there is a wealth of advanced sexual acts that may further enhance one's pleasure. Although not all of these will be to everyone's taste, having an understanding of deviations from the standard will help prepare scholars for anomalies they may encounter during field research, even if they are not prepared to entertain engaging in such practices. To advance to the next chapter, please ensure that you have:

- Identified the correct positions to use with non-optimal genital pairings
- Understood optimal techniques for traditional coital alignment
- Explored key advanced sexual positions (extra credit for field research)
- Developed a sexual position specifically designed for mutual satisfaction with your chosen study partner

Once this level of comprehension has been achieved, you may progress to coitus prohibitus, colloquially referred to as anal sex.

YOU MAY ALSO WISH TO CONSIDER USING AURAL OR VISUAL STIMULI TO HEIGHTEN THE EXPERIENCE OF COITUS, WHETHER IN THE FORM OF TALKING DIRTY, WATCHING AN ADULT VIDEO, OR READING EACH OTHER HIGHLIGHTS FROM EROTIC TEXTS.

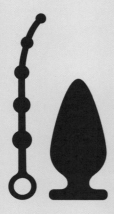

Chapter 6:
Coitus Prohibitus for the Fun of It

EXPLORING ANAL PLAY

Anal sex is still considered a taboo act by many. However, research indicates that it is becoming an increasingly common part of heterosexual couples' lives. While this may not seem controversial to the more adventurous scholar, the incidence of female to male anal coitus may be a little more surprising. According to a leading sex toy retailer, one-third of strap-on dildos sold are purchased by heterosexual couples to be used by the woman on the man.

Having a thorough understanding of the ways anal coitus can be most pleasurable is becoming increasingly more important. In addition, experiencing it in both the active and the passive positions is highly recommended for all serious students of the sexual arts.

ANAL SEX: A PRIMER

As mentioned earlier, the male has a prostate and the female does not. This means that anal sex is more likely to be highly pleasurable for the male than for the female. As such, strap-on sex is becoming increasingly common (see Female-to-Male Anal Coitus). Whether penetrating a male or a female anally, the basics remain the same.

As with all anal play, anal sex requires large amounts of lubricant. In addition, anal foreplay is essential (see chapter 3, A Better Hands-on Approach to Mating Rituals) to ensure that the sphincter is relaxed enough for comfortable access. It is also essential to wear a prophylactic to ensure that there is no transmission of diseases.

Once your partner is suitably receptive, lubricate the phallus (whether real or man-made) thoroughly and position it at the entrance of the anus. Do not push forward but, instead, allow your partner to grasp the phallus and refine the position to ensure that the angle of penetration is comfortable. At this point, the receiving partner should push back against the phallus, rather than having the giving partner push forward. Take it slowly, and pause to allow the anus to relax around the phallus at regular intervals.

When penetration reaches the maximum comfortable depth for the receiver, start thrusting in and out, but move slowly and keep the lubricant nearby to ensure the anus stays suitably well lubricated. Do not withdraw the phallus completely, or you'll need to start the entire process again because the anus tends to close up relatively quickly. Try to keep your movements smooth rather than jerky, and avoid speeding up unless your partner requests it or is clearly relaxed enough to enjoy rapid anal coitus.

You may choose to take anal sex to climax or use it as a form of foreplay. This should be dictated by the receiving partner, and anal coitus should stop immediately if there is any discomfort. Afterward, both parties should wash their hands and genitals to minimize the risk of infection.

MALE-TO-FEMALE ANAL COITUS

When entering into anal congress, a male may be tempted to ignore the rest of the body, particularly if anal sex is an act that he has fantasized about for years. However, it is important for the thoughtful student to consider his partner's pleasure.

Although women can undoubtedly gain stimulation though anal sex because of lateral stimulation of the G-spot, unlike in the male, there is no specific area inside the anus that brings sexual pleasure. As such, additional stimulation is recommended, not only to ensure mutual satisfaction, but also to help the woman—and her anus—remain relaxed.

Clitoral and breast stimulation are advisable unless both parties are used to anal coitus. Penetration of the vagina with a toy will tighten the anus, making penetration trickier. Try holding a bullet vibrator against the mons, clitoral hood, or clitoris, depending on your partner's clitoral sensitivity. Use lubricated fingers on the clitoris, being careful to use a different hand from the one used for anal stimulation, or stimulate the breasts with the hands or tongue.

If a degree of proficiency is attained in anal sex, you may wish to progress to using toys. However, ensure that you use soft rubber toys rather than hard plastic ones, or the tightness of the fit can cause the plastic to dig in, which adds a risk of vaginal or bladder bruising and can lead to cystitis.

Broaching the Taboo

Although anal sex is becoming increasingly common, many individuals may still have fears about the act. These concerns may play so heavily that the topic is ignored entirely, potentially limiting a couple from experimenting with an act that can be immensely satisfying.

Women may feel particularly uncomfortable about initiating a discussion of anal sex for fear that a curiosity may turn into an obligation. However, sophisticated scholars should be able to communicate clearly about all aspects of sex without committing to anything they do not wish to explore. Female scholars may also have concerns that they will be considered less than ladylike for wishing to engage in a taboo act. However, a well-balanced, confident, and mature male should have the mental capacity to take the information as it is intended. Indeed, any male who considers a woman to be a "slut" for clearly expressing a sexual desire is not a man with whom congress is to be advised.

Conversely, a male may feel as if he is pressuring his partner by raising the issue. He may have concerns that he'll be considered a "pervert" or may worry that his partner might doubt his sexuality. Again, these labels are negative, and education and enlightenment will provide the best foundation for appreciating the variety of human sexual expression. Enjoyment of anal sex and sexual preference are not linked, unless, of course, someone enjoys having anal sex with a partner of the same gender.

When raising the issue of anal coitus, the essential rule is to be honest and clear about your desires, expectations, and fears. You may find it easiest to write yourself notes first, to ensure that communication is open as possible. If taking this approach, however, do not leave the notes anywhere that an unaware partner could find them. This is most definitely a conversation to be had face to face.

Communicating while sober and without the influence of drugs is strongly advised. Liquid courage may be tempting, but it is likely to make the message ambiguous. Instead, share a romantic evening at home and wait for the topic of sex to reach its natural progression.

Rather than starting the conversation bluntly, initiate a discussion about whether there is anything sexual that your partner would like to try. This establishes a "safe" conversation zone in which sexual desires can be explored without putting your partner under pressure. From this point, it should be relatively easy to raise the issue of anal sex. Express your curiosity and allow your partner room to respond freely. If you are met with judgment, explain that you are not demanding the act but simply discussing it to learn whether it's something that you could experiment with together. If your partner is unwilling to try anal sex, but has an open-minded attitude, you could suggest lighter forms of anal play, such as fingering, rimming (but only ever with a dental dam), or anal toy play. If, however, your partner finds the entire area taboo, do not apply any pressure. Everyone has the right to decline an act that he or she finds distasteful. However, do not judge yourself harshly, or allow your partner to judge you harshly, for initiating the conversation. There is no shame to be had in wishing to explore sex to its fullest extent.

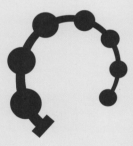

When it comes to penetration, it is advisable that the woman guide the phallus inside herself because the angle is all important. The woman should also set the pace, pushing back onto the penis as the anus relaxes. If anal sex is approached in this way, it is less likely to cause discomfort or anal tears, which makes it more likely that both parties will enjoy it and use it as a regular sexual practice.

FEMALE-TO-MALE ANAL COITUS

Although the use of strap-ons is still rare, an increasing amount of couples are discovering the joys of female-to-male anal coitus. This requires a female to wear a harness that has a dildo or vibrator attachment.

When purchasing a strap-on dildo, there are a few key considerations to bear in mind. First, the harness needs to fit. Harnesses come in many variations and can attach around the hips, thighs, or elsewhere.

Some harnesses have a built-in dildo. However, these are not recommended for novice students because they do not allow for gradually increasing the size of the toy over consecutive anal coitus sessions. Instead, it is better to opt for a harness that allows a variety of dildos to be attached. This gives the keen scholar the ability to start with a toy of relatively small dimensions and only increase the size as her partner sees fit.

When choosing a dildo for anal penetration, think carefully about the material that it is made from. The harder the material, the more difficult it is likely to be for a novice to take. Hard plastic and crystal should be avoided in favor of softer silicone or real-feel CyberSkin, which, as the name suggests, is designed to feel like the real thing.

Although the female scholar may be tempted to choose a toy that is of similar size to her partner's phallus on the basis that it will help him understand more clearly how anal sex feels to her, this should not be the starting position. Many males are particularly intimidated by anal penetration because they feel that it may call their masculinity into question. Greater education and a commitment to open-minded

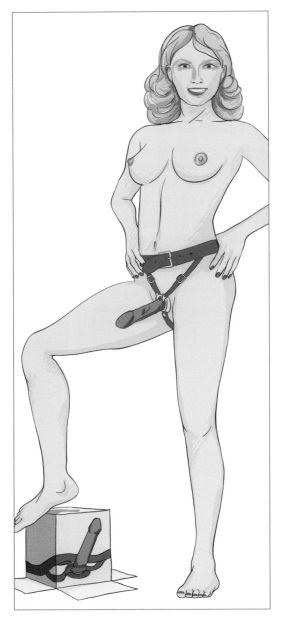

Figure 1: Many heterosexual couples are now experimenting with strap-on toys for anal penetration of the man.

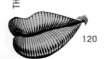

Anal Sizing

Unlike the vagina, the anus tends to be a similar size in most people. This plays no part in anal sex, however, because levels of anal relaxation vary from person to person. Some scholars may find it easy to relax, while others may find even the lightest circling of a finger causes the anus to contract.

A small amount of alcohol may ease relaxation. However, this also thins the blood, increasing the damage from any anal tears that may occur if the act does not go entirely as planned. This can happen despite both parties' best intentions and so should be treated as a cautionary tale.

By far the best way to relax the anus is to relax the mind. A sensual massage will help relieve tension, particularly if you ensure the buttocks get as much attention as the back. Some scholars have reported that erotic conversation helps set the mood, while others prefer to establish the pace so that the anus can open in its own time. Indeed, the nervous student could combine both approaches for maximum effect, assuming that "dirty talk" appeals to both partners.

Penis size is obviously a consideration in male-to-female anal sex. Although the anus can stretch, it is also prone to tearing. As such, it is inadvisable to attempt anal sex for the first time with a well-endowed man. Preparing the anus by using fingers and small toys before graduating to larger toys will help minimize the risk. This may take a matter of months.

Anal dilation kits are available, which help gradually stretch the anus. However, this is a major commitment, and there are horror stories about anal leaking after excessive stretching, so it is not something to be entered into lightly. It may be that a penis is simply too large to accommodate in this way. The male can still masturbate over the anus and rub the glans against it (wearing a condom to avoid infection), but penetration should always be at the receiving partner's behest.

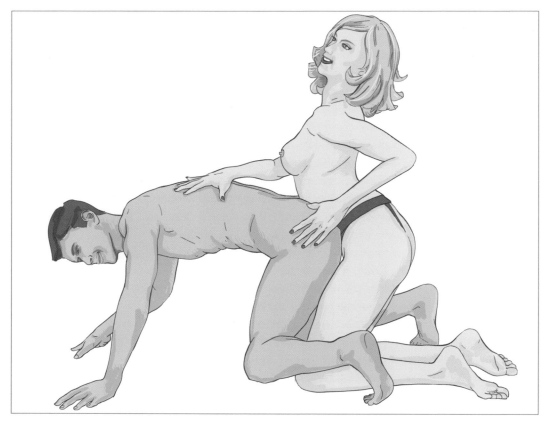

Figure 2: Go gently and use lots of lubricant when trying anal sex with a strap-on.

exploration should disabuse any such notions. Even so, if female-to-male anal sex is to become part of your sex life, it is best to introduce the topic gradually. Starting with a finger or a small pliable toy is more likely to garner a positive response. If using the finger, latex gloves are advised, both from a hygienic point of view and to ensure that any cuts on the fingers are not exposed to bacteria. Sexually transmitted infections can be passed through cuts, however small.

Vibrations will make a toy feel larger than it is. As such, vibrating toys should be avoided until the male has become sufficiently used to anal penetration to feel comfortable about pushing his limits.

The male should guide the dildo into himself because, unlike the penis, there is no feedback given by a dildo as to its location. Once the dildo has penetrated the anus, the female should allow the male to slowly push back onto it, rather than pushing forward herself, as a millimeter of extra depth can feel significantly larger when inside the anus. The male should not feel any pressure to speed the process: it is much easier to avoid accidental tearing of the sensitive anal skin if movements are extremely slow and well lubricated.

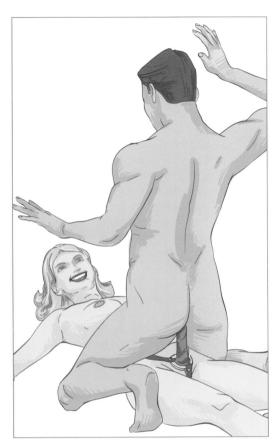

Figure 3: Being on top helps the receiving partner control the pace of anal sex.

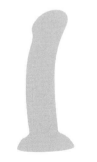

The female can masturbate the male as she penetrates him anally. However, some men are able to climax from prostate stimulation alone, often at surprising speed. As with male-to-female anal coitus, penetration should stop at the behest of the penetrated partner.

RECOMMENDED SEXUAL POSITIONS FOR ANAL SATISFACTION

While the lay scholar may assume that doggy-style is the only position for anal coitus, this is largely influenced by adult films, which are rarely indicative of optimal sexual practice. Ideally, the muscles surrounding the anus should be as relaxed as possible. As such, flat doggy is far preferable to standard doggy because it reduces tension in the thighs and buttocks.

Spooning offers a gentler approach to anal sex, which allows both parties the ability to control the proceedings. It also allows the male easy access to caress the female's clitoris and breasts.

Woman on top is ideal if a female is nervous about trying anal sex because it allows her to set the pace. This is also recommended if the male has a large penis, because it allows the female to control the depth of penetration.

Similarly, males may enjoy assuming the cowgirl or reverse cowgirl position to receive anal penetration. Reverse cowgirl is particularly beneficial because it allows the woman to masturbate the penis while penetrating the male from the rear.

Alternatively, the missionary position can be ideal for anal sex, though students new to anal coitus may find the positioning a little tricky at first. The initial complication is more than balanced by the enhanced sensation: females can enjoy clitoral stimulation as the male's torso rubs against the area, while males receiving anal coitus in this position can enjoy enhanced prostate stimulation due to the angle of entry.

TO DOUCHE OR NOT TO DOUCHE?

Although adult stars tend to douche before anal coitus as a matter of course, this is not required for recreational anal sex. It is done purely to ensure that visual integrity is maintained throughout the anal coitus scene. However, there is minimal risk of fecal matter being in the rectum if you have a healthy diet: it generally stays farther up the digestive system. Regular anal douching can lead the rectum to dry out and tear, weaken natural defenses, and cause constipation. Despite introducing water into the area, anal douching actually dehydrates the colon. As an added warning, some people become dependent on enemas to evacuate their bowels after regular use. Therefore, it's not to be recommended.

That said, some people feel self-conscious about entering into anal play without "cleaning up" first. This is best done by wiping thoroughly with a specially designed intimate wipe, avoiding eating for a few hours before sex, and filling an ear syringe with warm water to squirt into the anus and then release. This should clean the area adequately for anal play.

If you insist on douching the anus despite the risks, do ensure that you use a specially designed enema kit. This generally includes a hot water bottle–style bag, with a hook to hang it up, attached to a hose with a nozzle.

Before use, ensure that you have emptied your bowels to minimize the work required by the enema kit. Fill the bag with warm water. Cold water can cause painful cramping, and soap or any other additives may lead to inflammation, so use nothing but warm water in the bag.

The bag will generally contain about 2 liters (2 quarts) of liquid. This should be introduced into the anus by means of the nozzle attached to the hose, after which point you should try to hold the water inside your rectum for around twenty minutes. If it feels too uncomfortable, do not try to force more water inside yourself or endeavor to hold the water in. Some cramping is to be expected, but pain is the body's way of telling you that you are doing something wrong.

Ensure that you are sitting on the toilet when administering the enema as it is an unusual sensation and liquid is liable to leak out. Once you have held the water inside you, expel it in the usual fashion. After the water is expelled, you may feel the urge to defecate again, in which case do so. Afterward, you may choose to repeat the process or may deem yourself clean enough. Given the risks, the less you douche, the better.

Note: Do not douche immediately before anal coitus because it is not unusual for some water to be retained inside the colon. This may lead to a messier experience than anal coitus with no prior douching. Instead, wait at least eight hours to give your body the opportunity to expel any excess water.

UTILIZING PSYCHOLOGY FOR OPTIMAL ANAL PLAY

As with vaginal coitus, the success of anal coitus can be affected by a partner's sexual psychology. A submissive partner is more likely to enjoy vehement anal coitus, while a dominant partner may not wish to entertain the idea at all. That said, it is possible to come up with scenarios in which one partner may retain dominance over the other while receiving anal penetration (for example, telling the partner administering anal sex that this is the only part of the penetrated partner that she deserves).

It is also perfectly possible to have tender and loving anal coitus. This mood can be enhanced by sharing a sensual bath or shower together prior to anal congress, and massaging the receiving partner once climax has been reached.

Because anal sex encourages the body to produce painkilling endorphins, it may lead to a "come down" in which the penetrated partner feels tearful afterward. If so, this is easily dealt with by being particularly affectionate toward said partner, wrapping him up warmly, and running him a relaxing bath if the feeling does not pass within around ten minutes.

Generally speaking, anal coitus should draw a couple closer, regardless of which gender is being penetrated, as it shows a deep level of intimacy that can increase the loving bond between mates.

ANALYZING AND HONING THE EFFECTIVENESS OF YOUR APPROACH

After successful coitus prohibitus, scholars may feel that they have achieved the pinnacle of sexual knowledge. However, before graduation can be achieved, it is worth gaining an understanding of issues that may negatively impact mating in general. Only when the student feels able to cope with any sexual situation can true mastery of the subject area be claimed.

To advance to the next chapter, please ensure that you have:

- Learned how to correctly prepare for anal coitus
- Understood the basics of anal coitus
- Explored anal coitus in both the passive and the active role
- Discovered your ideal positions for both giving and receiving anal coitus

Once this level of comprehension has being achieved, you may progress to learning about common issues in the field.

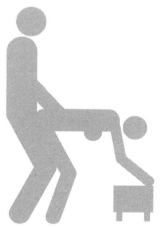

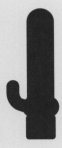

Chapter 7:

Overcoming Common Issues in the Field

TROUBLESHOOTING TECHNIQUES FOR COMMON SEXUAL PROBLEMS

After experiencing the myriad joys of manual, oral, genital, and anal coitus, neophyte students are likely to feel secure in their knowledge. However, problems in the field offer the greatest scope for learning. Until you are able to deal with any sexual issues that may arise with style and grace, there is no way you can attain the ultimate qualification.

Common sexual problems are nothing to fear. Human sexual response is complex, and so it should come as no surprise that sometimes events do not go as planned (see *The Issue-Free Sex Life: Celibacy in Contemporary Culture*, by Dr. Noah Chung).

PREMATURE EJACULATION

Most men experience premature ejaculation at some point in their lives, whether as a reaction to extreme stimulation or simply because they have not yet mastered full control of their sexual arousal. It is important for male students to realize that, while premature ejaculation may be crushing to the male sense of self-esteem, it offers a boost to the female ego. By playing on this aspect, emphasizing the beauty and sexual charm of one's mate, a negative can be turned into a positive. However, should ejaculation limit further congress, it is only fair to ensure the female is pleasured in an alternative way, rather than simply assuming that coitus stops at the point of male ejaculation.

If the problem is ongoing, the sufferer should seek advice from a physician, as there may be a medical or psychological reason that is the cause. If, however, it is a relatively rare occurrence, a few tricks and techniques will help.

Nowadays, there are numerous delay prophylactics available. These are coated with a numbing anesthetic that helps diminish the level of stimulation received by the male without affecting the female's pleasure. All women should ensure that they have these condoms on hand, along with regular, extra-large, and stimulating condoms, to ensure that all situations can be dealt with. It is best to keep these in a discreet condom case, as males may feel intimidated if presented with an array of prophylactics, particularly if any option other than "extra large" is chosen. In addition, this will prevent strangers from approaching you with undignified requests should you drop your handbag and scatter the contents on the floor (see *Me Stud, You Slut: Neanderthal Sexual Attitudes Explored*, by Ms. Andrist).

Males can reduce the incidence of premature ejaculation by practicing controlling sexual response during masturbation. As climax approaches, the male should stop self-stimulation and allow the penis to soften slightly before resuming masturbation. With practice, this method of masturbation can help extend the amount of time that a male can last during coitus. In addition, it offers the ideal excuse should a partner catch a male scholar masturbating when he has promised to do the dishes, on the basis that the indulgence is selfless, done purely with the objective of improving the female's pleasure. Please note that this line is only likely to work once.

Kegel exercises will also help a male last longer during sex, as strong PC muscles will help enhance ejaculatory control. Do a minimum of ten repetitions per day, every day, to help build stronger muscles. Ensure the door is locked, as being caught with a towel draped over the penis as one raises and lowers it is liable to cause hilarity.

During sex, focus on shallow penetration rather than deep thrusts, as these tend to offer less stimulation. Pressing the penis against the female's G-spot rather than penetrating more vigorously will pleasure the female (assuming that she enjoys G-spot stimulation) without speeding orgasm excessively. In addition, Kegel flexes while penetrating the female may boost her pleasure and still allow the male to maintain control.

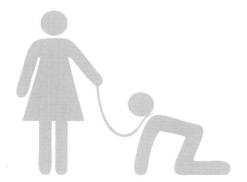

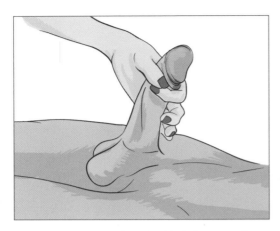

Figure 1: Never stop experimenting. It's the best way to learn.

Sex experts William Masters and Virginia Johnson recommend the "squeeze technique" to delay ejaculation. This entails applying firm pressure to the penis with the thumb and forefinger, focusing pressure on the urethra. Given the sensitivity of the area, this is best done by the male. Under no circumstances should a female utilize this technique without warning (see *Reader, I Broke Him: A Cautionary Tale*, by Anonymous).

The female can help by paying close attention to her lover's responses and pulling away or changing position or technique should climax seem imminent. Talking may also help distract the partner from climax, though both the erotic and the mundane should be avoided: instead, try saying, "Can we change position?" or "I love you," as neither is likely to elicit immediate climax and both will help distract the male from the physical sensations that could otherwise lead to ejaculation. It should also be noted that talking during sex will delay climax in a male who does not suffer from premature ejaculation.

Further, both parties should ensure that the female is close to climax at the moment of penetration. This will increase the likelihood of both partners reaching orgasm during coitus.

WAIT FOR IT: DELAYED EJACULATION

Conversely, many males suffer from delayed ejaculation. This is a common side effect of certain medications, including many antidepressants. In addition, stress, nervousness, tiredness, alcohol, and recreational drugs can cause delayed climax. As such, this condition tends to affect a vast number of men at some point in their lives.

If the female scholar is approached by a male in a state of inebriation or under the influence of drugs, it is best to avoid congress, not only because the risk of delayed ejaculation is high, but also because the experience is likely to be lacking in fulfillment. Further, it is unlikely that the male will be able to accurately gauge his true levels of attraction toward the female (see *Beyond the Beer Goggles: An Analysis of Morning-After Misery*, by Dr. Neve Agayne).

If, however, the problem becomes apparent in a sober man once sexual contact has been initiated, there are various approaches to take. First, do not draw attention to the issue. While honesty is an important part of sexual communication, knowing when to stay silent is equally important. Additional stress is only likely to heighten the problem. Instead, you have various options.

You can employ the techniques recommended for an insensitive or highly insensitive penis in the oral-genital and manual stimulation chapters of this book. Remember that lubricant is essential for prolonged stimulation of the genital region to guard against chafing.

Alternatively, you can take a more cerebral approach and distract the male from the issue at hand by reading him an erotic story or watching an adult film together. Should you lack access to either of these, a striptease or masturbation show can have a similar, if not more intense, effect.

And of course, there's no reason that congress has to conclude with climax for both parties. While it is desirable, in general, for both the male and the female

ABOVE ALL, THE FEMALE SHOULD ENSURE THAT SHE MAINTAINS A HEALTHY SENSE OF SELF-ESTEEM. DELAYED EJACULATION IS NO INDICATION THAT A PARTNER HAS LOST DESIRE: IT'S SIMPLY A SYMPTOM OF MODERN LIFE.

to reach climax, joy can also be gained through selflessly pleasuring a partner. If male ejaculation seems unlikely, it is the optimum time to ask for a massage, as the gentleman is more likely to focus on the job at hand rather than prodding the female in the back with an engorged member.

Above all, the female should ensure that she maintains a healthy sense of self-esteem. Delayed ejaculation is no indication that a partner has lost desire: it's simply a symptom of modern life.

THE ELUSIVE FEMALE ORGASM

Many women also have orgasmic issues on occasion, again as a result of excessive drinking or drug use, side effects from certain medications, an unhealthy lifestyle, stress, or insecurity. This is not the same as a woman taking longer to reach climax than a male through penetrative sex, a problem that is generally easily rectified by ensuring there is at least twenty minutes of foreplay prior to initiating coitus. As with men, modern life can take its toll on the female.

Again, it is worth utilizing techniques recommended for an insensitive or highly insensitive clitoris. Sex toys can prove particularly useful due to the intensity of the stimulation, especially when controlled by the female. An erotic massage may help relax a stressed partner, thus improving the chances of climax. And stimulating the brain with an erotic story or adult film can work equally well with women as with men. Dirty talk can also prove highly effective, as women tend to be more linguistically aroused than men.

Removing the pressure to climax may help. There is nothing wrong with having the occasional session of coitus in which only one partner climaxes, as long as it's not a regular occurrence because this may lead to resentment. Indeed, a fantasy element can be incorporated to turn a negative into a positive: the male can "ban" the female from climaxing and order her to pleasure him instead (obviously, this role-play can be reversed in cases of delayed ejaculation).

It is worth noting that sexual response in both genders tends to be significantly higher when a healthy lifestyle is maintained. Layers of fat caused by obesity may limit nerve response and, indeed, shrink the apparent size of the penis or visibility of the clitoris. Alcohol is commonly known to provoke desire and, at the same time, lessen performance; smoking limits blood flow, which can slow engorgement of the genitals; and while recreational drugs may seem appealing, most hamper sexual response or, at the very least, recall of the event. Lack of sleep can affect not only sexual arousal but also mood, increasing the risk of petty annoyances developing into arguments and thus decreasing the chances of coitus being initiated. The keen scholar should ensure that the body is kept fit to maximize the chances of pleasurable coupling.

WHO ARE YOU CALLING A PERVERT?: CONFLICTING SEXUAL FANTASIES

In addition to understanding the physical issues that may arise, dedicated students should ensure that they can cope with a clash of sexual fantasies or levels of physical desire. Although thorough fieldwork prior to sexual congress is one of the best ways to guard against a mismatch, even the most ardent scholar may rush into coitus when confronted with a seemingly ultimately desirable mate.

Should a partner raise a fantasy or desire that you find amusing, under no circumstances should you laugh. Balloon fetishes, "sploshing" (in which partners cover each other in food, have whipped cream pie fights, and generally get messy), and furryism (in which people wear giant furry animal costumes) are all established fetishes and should not be treated with any more scorn than the more common fetishes, such as a penchant for stockings or high heels.

SHOULD A PARTNER RAISE A FANTASY
OR DESIRE THAT YOU FIND AMUSING,
UNDER NO CIRCUMSTANCES
SHOULD YOU LAUGH.

Instead, aim to understand the fantasy better by asking your mate when the fantasy first became appealing, what it is that makes it such an attractive idea, and whether there are any milder variations that could offer similar stimulation. Willingness to compromise is an essential part of being a good lover, though if every sexual encounter requires compromise it may be worth examining whether the relationship is truly an ideal match.

Should the desire be something that you could never consider doing, explain your reasoning without judgment: declining a sex act because it is "weird" is unfair. A partner is showing trust and honesty by admitting to a secret desire and responding negatively is punishing this positive behavior. Instead, focus on physical or mental blockages that stop you from finding the idea arousing. For example, if a mate indicates an interest in anal coitus but you find it distasteful, consider whether it is due to concerns about hygiene, self-consciousness about being touched in such an intimate place, or a sign of subconscious (or indeed, conscious) homophobia. By discussing the issues that underlie your unwillingness to comply with your partner's desire, you may find yourself becoming more open-minded about exploring new things—though no one should ever feel pressured into trying anything sexual against his or her will.

If, however, the fantasy or desire is something that is merely surprising, rather than actively unappealing, consider trying it. Only through experiencing something can you gauge an accurate measure of whether it is an activity that you enjoy. Many students have been pleasantly surprised to discover that an idea they initially found amusing offers a great deal of sexual satisfaction. The sexual scholar should be open to new ideas.

ANALYZING AND HONING THE EFFECTIVENESS OF YOUR APPROACH

By now, the scholar should be feeling confident enough to face almost all sexual situations and deal with any issues that may arise with grace and charm. However, for total mastery of the sexual arena, it is worth covering a few of the more unusual quirks that may be encountered in the field.

To advance to the next chapter, please ensure that you have:

- Learned how to deal with premature ejaculation
- Understood coping mechanisms for delayed ejaculation
- Developed suitable skills to work around elusive orgasm in the female
- Gained comprehension in dealing with conflicting sexual desires

Once this level of understanding has been achieved, you may progress to the final chapter, Advanced Studies for the Impassioned Student.

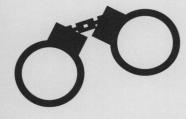

Chapter 8:

Advanced Studies for the Impassioned Student

FETISHISTIC BEHAVIORS TO ENHANCE SEXUAL VARIETY

By utilizing all the techniques that have been detailed up to this point, the sexual scholar can gain thorough sexual satisfaction. However, should additional stimulation be required, the field of fetishism offers a great range of sexual seasonings that can further enhance the experience. Everyone has a penchant for different experiences. It is likely that some fetishes will have more appeal than others, and indeed, some may leave you cold. There is no reason to explore all fetishes any more than there is a reason to enter into coitus with everyone you meet. However, the information in this chapter offers a "shopping list" that is designed to help you identify your niche sexual preferences.

ADULT ENGAGEMENT IN THE GAME OF DOCTOR AND NURSE

This subject covers a hugely diverse area. Although everyone's fantasies are different, there are some that are particularly common (see boxes). Although fantasy exploration can be highly enjoyable, it is best explored after a relationship has become established. Fantasies can be highly compelling and, as such, if you engage in fantasy play before all standard routes have been explored, it can minimize the impact of oral, manual-genital, and genital contact without a fantasy element. Given that this early exploration is likely to form the basis of your long-term sexual relationship, it should be given due care and attention rather than sped through in a hasty desire to progress to more extreme behavior.

The best way to explore fantasies is by taking turns in confessing a desire, starting with the mildest fantasies and only progressing to more extreme fantasies if you receive a positive response. Exchanging fantasies with your partner helps limit

TOP FEMALE SEXUAL FANTASIES

Fantasies about their partner	**21%**
Group sex	**15%**
Sex in a romantic or an exotic setting	**15%**
Rape/force	**13%**
No fantasies at all	**12%**
Identified people (other than partner)	**8%**
Voyeurism/fetishism	**7%**
Sadomasochism	**7%**

(Source: Glenn Wilson, *The Great Sex Divide* [Washington, DC: Scott-Townsend, 1992], pp. 10–14.)

potential judgment, as almost everyone has at least one desire that might be considered extreme by another party. Conversely, do not laugh at a partner for sharing a fantasy that does nothing for you. Simply accept that everyone is different and, if the idea does not appeal, state this in a nonjudgmental way. Even if you are not prepared to entertain a fantasy, it is worth considering talking dirty to your partner about his or her desires because this shows a willingness to accept a partner without pushing your own parameters to uncomfortable levels.

If you decide to live out a fantasy, go slowly and ensure you have a safe word in place. This is a word that is not used in standard sexual congress and means "stop immediately." The "traffic light" system is common, in which red is used to indicate a desire to stop, yellow to slow down, and green to progress once more. However, you can use any word of your choice. Avoid "no" or "stop," as these words may be used in fantasy play (for example, in a pirate and captor situation) and may send a mixed message.

TOP MALE SEXUAL FANTASIES

Fantasy	Percentage
Group sex	31%
Voyeurism/fetishism	18%
Fantasies about their partner	14%
Identified people (other than partner)	8%
Sadomasochism	7%
No fantasies at all	5%
Sex in a romantic or an exotic setting	4%
Rape/force	4%
Everything	3%

(Source: Glenn Wilson, *The Great Sex Divide* [Washington, DC: Scott-Townsend, 1992], pp. 10–14.)

You can also enhance fantasies with the use of outfits. Although there are numerous costumes available online, it is easy to tailor your wardrobe to devise erotic attire with very little expenditure.

A black dress can become a French maid's outfit with the addition of a white apron and frilly cap; a seductive spy or a high-class escort with the addition of high heels, stockings, and maybe a hidden sex toy or pair of handcuffs; or a stern dominatrix with the addition of high boots and a riding crop.

Conversely, a black suit can be turned into a James Bond outfit with the addition of a martini glass and hidden sex toys; a glamorous photographer with the addition of a black turtleneck and maybe a beret; or a stern boss, ready to punish his secretary for her poor dictation skills.

A little imagination is all that is needed to incorporate fantasy into your sex life. Scholars should be aware that role-playing with a partner may lead one or both of you to laugh at some point. However, this is nothing to fear: if you laugh together rather than at each other, it can lead to greater intimacy and help strengthen the bond between you.

UTILIZING BUTTOCK STRIKING TO REACH SEXUAL NIRVANA

Although basic spanking can be incorporated into standard sex play (see chapter 3, A Better Hands-on Approach to Mating Rituals), some people have a stronger attraction to the act than can be satisfied with a playful slap. If so, it may be worth experimenting with more advanced spanking techniques.

The position a person is in while a spanking is administered can have a huge psychological effect on the experience. Pulling a lover over one's knee can conjure up images of the lord of the manor and his wanton wench, or a naughty student who hasn't done his homework. Standing with the arms bound above the head while being spanked can evoke images of being captured by pirates or arrested by a corrupt police officer. And kneeling on all fours can be

particularly humiliating, and is apt if you are exploring a master/mistress and slave scenario. Again, ensure that a safe word is in place before commencing this kind of activity.

Should you find that your hands hurt from administering a spanking, leather gloves will help reduce the sting. Alternatively, spanking paddles may be incorporated to add extra levels of pain. However, as with manual spanking, the initial strokes should be gentle to allow the body to release endorphins before progressing to firmer strokes. There are spanking paddles of various kinds, made from leather or wood, covered with velvet or fake fur; you can even get spanking paddles that leave a heart shape or the imprint of a word such as "slut" on a partner's bottom, or it could lead to humiliation of an entirely nonerotic variety.

It is particularly important to tend to your lover's buttocks after a hard spanking has been administered to ensure there is no lasting discomfort. Rubbing body lotion designed for sensitive skin on the area will help ease the pain. For a kinky twist, you might decide to dust the buttocks with talcum powder, lick your finger, and "sign your work." Taking a photograph of this (with your lover's consent) can then give you a fond memory in pictorial form to enjoy.

ASSUME THE POSITION: ADVANCED CONSENSUAL CORPORAL PUNISHMENT

Although the basics of whipping are akin to spanking in that it revolves around endorphin release through the induction of mild pain, the technique is very different. Whipping can be extreme, but it can also be highly sensual.

Beginners may find that a suede cat-o'-nine-tails-style whip offers the broadest range of possibilities. The soft fronds can be gently trailed over the primary and secondary erogenous regions, while a mild sting can be delivered by circling the whip, causing the fronds to softly whip the buttocks or breasts. It can take a little time to master the technique. Try

Introducing Third Parties into Coitus

The adventurous scholar may be tempted to introduce multiple partners into the equation once a thorough understanding of mutual coitus has been gained. However, such are the complexities of the ménage à trois that it would require another volume to fully comprehend the topic.

There are two types of (broadly) heterosexual threesomes: FFM (two females and one male) and MMF (two males and one female). The former offers additional breasts and orifices for the male to explore. In addition, males may enjoy feeling two pairs of lips pleasuring their phallus, and the extra hands can be used for many different forms of stimulation.

However, unless the women have Sapphic inclinations, all but the most stamina-filled male will find the experience exhausting, and it is likely that one or both females will remain unsatisfied by the experience. In addition, males are often inclined to focus purely on the physical, forgetting that two women mean twice the amount of conversation will be required. Some scholars may consider this price too high to pay.

The latter scenario offers dual-penetration options, namely, DP (dual penetration of the vagina and anus) and "spit-roasting" (dual penetration of the mouth and vagina or, less commonly, anus). While an MMF threesome offers the female a greater opportunity for satisfaction, she should be aware that male insecurities about genital size can have a considerable negative bearing, particularly if there is a significant difference in penile stature. Further, a female who is not inclined toward anal coitus may find herself declining tediously repetitive requests due to the common incidence of DP in adult films.

Should you wish to enter into group coitus, it is wise to do so without the complications of existing relationships, whether sexual or merely friendships. It should go without saying that safe sex is a must, but given that group sex is often initiated after consumption of excessive amounts of alcohol, the reminder is valid.

practicing rotating the flogger in figure eights that are the same size and shape of the buttocks; using a cushion rather than your partner's derriere is advisable until a basic mastery has been gained.

A leather whip will offer a middle ground, as it has reasonable amounts of give but can still be wielded gently. Avoid leather whips with studs or knots unless you are looking for an intensely painful toy.

For a more thorough punishment, a leather crop works well, and it is also a good way of working up to a cane. However, do not use the full length of the crop: only hit your partner with the end, as this delivers an impressive noise with a comparatively mild sting.

Canes offer a fiercer sting, and are more inclined to leave bruises or break the skin. As such, they are not ideal for beginners but can invoke a highly charged response in a partner who enjoys pain and pleasure being combined. They should be used in a similar way to spanking paddles, with initial lighter strokes used to provoke endorphin release before progressing to more intense stinging strokes.

Note: Care should be taken to ensure that the crop, cane, or flogger does not hit the eyes, and, as with spanking, the lower back should be avoided to limit risk of kidney damage. Any toy that breaks the skin or is used for genital contact should be used solely with one partner, as the natural fabrics that most whips and canes are made from are difficult to clean and there is a risk of transmitting blood-borne infections if whips and canes are shared. If whipping is something that forms a regular part of your sex life, it is worth investing in a guide that is specifically designed to educate students about this practice, as there are many nuances that can be explored within the art.

WATCH AND LEARN: A PORNOGRAPHY PRIMER

Such is the availability of pornography that any student who has progressed to this stage in the program is sure to have a thorough awareness of its infinite variety. However, as a brief summary, pornography is available in written, pictorial, and video form, and is primarily distributed online in the current climate. Every taste and inclination is catered to, though scholars are not advised to test this premise to exhaustion, as there are no limits as to what you may see.

User-generated pornography is becoming increasingly common. Should you choose to indulge your exhibitionistic fantasies in this way, ensure that your face and any identifiable piercings or tattoos are hidden. If not, you can guarantee that your potential future dream employer will encounter the video, thus denying your chances of career success (or at least ensuring your chances of extreme embarrassment). No matter how drunk you are, resist the urge to label the video with your real name. When broaching the subject of pornography, tread carefully, as many people object to its existence. However, those who question the ethics of its existence should be aware of the strong feminist porn movement, which allows arousal without objectification. Ideally, choose an adult video online with your lover to ensure that you select one that will appeal to you both.

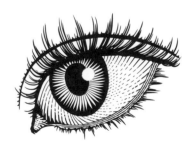

A MECHANIZED WORLD: EROTIC AND ROBOTIC TOYS

In addition to the standard toys detailed in earlier chapters, there are numerous extreme machines on the market. These include sex swings that allow you to position a partner as you see fit; sex machines that allow one or both parties to engage in full coitus with an artificial penis or vagina that genuinely thrusts or flexes; and electro-stimulating devices, in which safe levels of electric current can be passed through a lover's erogenous zones (though never above the heart, as this can be lethal).

There are also more bizarre toys such as the Space Hopper dildo, which allows you to bounce up and down while being penetrated; the dildo pogo stick, which is exactly as the name suggests; and the Real Doll, an anatomically correct doll that can be tailored to your exact specifications, from pubic hair style to eye color, and is available in both male and female models.

Indeed, we are rapidly reaching a time when robotic sexual companions could become the norm. A sex robot named Roxxxy was unveiled at the 2010 AVN Show (an annual gathering for the adult trade industry). Programmed with artificial intelligence, the robot allows users to choose from a variety of personalities, including "Frigid Farrah" and "Wild Wendy," in addition to customizing her look. Exactly why one would wish to have a frigid sex robot remains unexplained (though it could relate to the popularity of "the girlfriend experience" within the sex worker trade, in which men pay for a prostitute to behave as if she were his girlfriend, albeit generally of the more welcoming variety).

Tailoring Fetishes to Genital Differences

Although fetishes are primarily driven by cognition, they can also be used to assist with genital mismatches.

If a woman finds penetration difficult, for example, exploring alternate forms of arousal is recommended. Spanking, role-play, voyeurism, or exhibitionism may all offer stimulation.

If a female has a highly sensitive clitoris, playing orgasm-denial games, in which every inch of the body is stimulated except the genital region and clitoral contact has to be begged for by the female, may offer a heated way to tackle the issue.

Should a woman have a loose vagina, penetration with multiple toys may appeal. Should the female have submissive yearnings, this can be teamed with bondage. Receiving anal sex while being tied up may appeal to the more extreme submissive.

In addition to offering conversation, Roxxxy provides fully functional orifices that are always available. However, at $9,000, robotic sexual companions are a niche market, giving plenty of time to ponder the ethical implications of their existence in terms of female objectification.

Robots aside, as with standard sex toys, by far the best way to choose a toy to enjoy together is to visit a sex toy website online and have a full and frank discussion about which toys appeal. Do ensure that you start at the milder end of the scale, however; a new partner may feel nervous about spending the night with a violet wand and a real doll replica of him- or herself—and indeed, even in a long-term relationship you may find that some toys are simply beyond the pale.

ANALYZING AND HONING THE EFFECTIVENESS OF YOUR APPROACH

After successfully studying all sections of this book, the hardworking scholar will possess the knowledge to gracefully tackle any sexual situation, having gained a thorough understanding of one's own genital structures and those of the opposite gender.

Any anomalies encountered in the field, whether physical or psychological, will be easily taken in the student's stride. Scholars will know how to identify and approach a suitable mate, pleasure said mate through stimulation of the primary and secondary erogenous zones, and approach all types of coitus in a confident and informed manner.

The student's sexual toy box will be thoroughly equipped with all the tools required to provide myriad forms of pleasure. Alternative practices will have been considered and, ideally, explored, and fantasies will have been shared with a partner, assuming the relationship is at the appropriate stage.

In short, the student will be a sexual encyclopedia, keen to share knowledge with an appropriate partner and willing to learn more with every new encounter. Once this level of comprehension has been achieved, your studies are complete. Congratulations. You are a Bachelor of the Field (BoF). Enjoy.

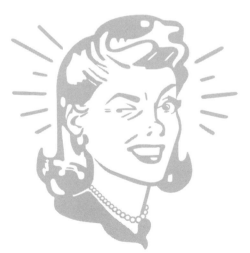

Certificate of Graduation

I, the undersigned, do solemnly swear that I have read and thoroughly absorbed *The Field Guide to F*cking* and undertaken all practical assessments included in the guide.

Name: _____

Signature: _____

The above candidate has fulfilled all criteria to progress to qualified research in the field, having gained a thorough understanding of coitus and associated acts.

This certificate is proof of your Bachelor of the Field award.
[Signature of Examining Board]

Resources

The ardent scholar may want continue studying once the initial qualification has been gained. The following resources may prove useful in this objective. All sex toys and products mentioned in this volume, with the exception of niche items such as the robotic sex doll, are available from the websites listed below. The remaining products can easily be found through an Internet search.

WEBSITES

Adultfriendfinder.com Contact website that offers the opportunity for in-depth analysis of the many sexual subcultures that may be encountered in the field. The site can also help students to meet study partners, particularly those into more niche pleasures.

Babeland.com Excellent U.S-based, sex-positive erotic emporium, with a diverse array of products presented in a tasteful way.

Cliterati.co.uk Erotic website created by this book's author, offering thousands of user-generated sexual fantasies categorized into straight, gay, sub/dom, group, and taboo (for more niche fetishes). Students may wish to add a story to gain extra credits. All content is free to access.

Femplay.co.uk/au Australian erotic emporium designed with a female audience in mind, offering sex toys, pubic shavers, and numerous kinky accessories.

Fetteredpleasures.com Bondage and fetish website selling whips, chains, fetish clothing, pony and puppy play accessories, plus items that even the most devoted scholar may need to research before understanding the designated use.

Ifeelmyself.com Both educational and erotic, this site offers user-generated art videos of people—primarily female—indulging in the act of self-pleasure.

JanesGuide.com An excellent website offering balanced reviews of online erotic material.

Sexplained.com An educational website that offers advice about safe sex and sexually transmitted infections.

SheSaidBoutique.com United Kingdom–based designer erotic boutique offering premium corsets, designer toys, and kinky treats.

Scarleteen.com Advice on sexual health, sexuality, and sexual politics for teenagers but equally informative for adult scholars.

Tickledonline.co.uk Sex advice combined with an array of the latest toys for couples of all sexualities. It also offers numerous online erotic resources for the neophyte scholar.

BOOKS
FICTION
***Delta of Venus*, Anaïs Nin** Erotic short stories of a literary—and occasionally shocking—nature.

***Justine*, Marquis de Sade** One of de Sade's most infamous books, it follows the particularly cruel enslavement of the female in the titular role.

***The Story of O*, Pauline Reage** This sadomasochistic classic is rumored to have been written as a series of love letters. It offers valuable insight into the fetish scene, focusing on the willing acquiescence of a female slave, and is sure to be erotically charged for those with an interest in such matters.

***Venus in Furs*, Leopold von Sacher-Masoch** For those whose penchant for fetish errs on the side of male domination, Masoch's classic erotic novel examines the treatment of a male slave by his cruel mistress.

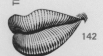

Vox, **Nicholson Baker** Erotic odyssey exploring an array of creative sexual fantasies in a literary and contemporary way. The creativity becomes particularly apparent during a memorable scene with a paint roller.

NONFICTION

Erotic Home Video: Create Your Own Adult Films, **Anna Span** A well-informed and easy-to-follow guide to erotic filmmaking from Europe's leading female porn producer and director.

Guide To Getting It On, **Paul Joannides** This is a great primer for students who feel need additional support to fully comprehend the complexities of coitus.

My Secret Garden, **Nancy Friday** Nancy Friday's first book created the concept of female sexual fantasies. In 1973, this was deemed extremely shocking. However, her impressive research ensured that female sexual fantasy became an acceptable part of both academic research and media coverage of sexual matters. Friday's later books covered topics that included male sexual fantasy and jealousy. These offer the keen scholar valuable insight into sexuality. Less devoted students may find titillation in the fantasies that formed the basis of Friday's research and are included in the book.

The Big Bang, **Em and Lo** (Emma Taylor and Lorelei Sharke) This informative book offers an insight into almost every sexual practice, explaining how to experiment safely, deal with common hazards, and generally become a better lover. Students may particularly appreciate the lighthearted tone.

The Anal Sex Position Guide, **Tristan Taormino** Quite possibly the world's leading expert in anal sex, Taormino explains the ins and outs of anal sex with élan. Showing that there is a plethora of anal sex choice, Taormino's informed and honest advice is presented in an accessible and entertaining way.

Acknowledgments

Thanks, as ever, to my amazing agent Chelsey Fox of Fox and Howard and the lovely folks at Quiver—publisher William Kiester, acquisitions editor Jill Alexander, and developmental editor Cara Connors—for helping me develop and hone this book from its inception to the finished product you hold in your hands right now.

Thanks to my dad, Jason Goss, my stepmum, Heather Kesterton, my mum, Jean Dubberley, and my sisters, Juliet Dubberley and Becky Goss, for being loving, kind, creative people who have always supported my choices—and allowed me the room to make (and learn from) my own mistakes. I love you.

Thanks to Tom Rea for thoughtfully providing me with a wonderful writing desk, valuable field research, and insightful ideas. He'll know what I mean when I say, "Fuck off."

Most of all, thanks to you for buying this book. I hope that it helps you enjoy the field in the way that suits you best.

About the Author

EMILY DUBBERLEY is the author of numerous books, including *Things a Woman Should Know About Seduction*, *Sex Play*, *Friendly Fetish*, and *I'd Rather Be Single Than Settle*. Her books have sold more than a million copies worldwide.

She is frequently quoted as an expert in magazines, including *Cosmopolitan*, *Elle*, and *Company* and has written for numerous publications, including *Grazia*, *FHM*, *Elle*, and *Men's Health*, and has had articles syndicated worldwide. She's written for and appeared on television shows in Canada and the United Kingdom, including the *Joan Rivers Position* on British Channel 5, and she writes for numerous websites, including iVillage.co.uk and msn.com.

After graduating with a social psychology degree, specializing in sexuality, she was short-listed for the *Cosmopolitan* Journalism Scholarship, and the *Company* Fiction Writer Award. She founded cliterati.co.uk in 2001, an online women's magazine. It has attracted more than half a million page impressions per month and international press coverage.

She created Burlesque Against Breast Cancer, burlesqueabc.com, and the books, *Ultimate Burlesque* and *Ultimate Decadence*, all to raise money for Macmillan Cancer Support. To date, they have raised more than $23,000 (£15,000 U.K.) and inspired international events.

She founded the magazines *Lovers' Guide*, *Scarlet*, and *EK*. She wrote the five most recent *Lovers' Guide* videos, edited the *Lovers' Guide* magazine, and helped create loversguide.com.

She has written for brands, including Philips Satinelle, Schloer, and Trojan Condoms, and has been a consultant on campaigns for brands, including Ann Summers, Gumtree, sextoys.co.uk, and Virgin Megastores.

Her latest projects are groweatgift.com, a guide to gardening that's aimed at a sophisticated urban audience, and forestofthoughts.co.uk, an organization that exists to promote science and arts events and collaborations. She lives in England.